Free From Menopause In 6 Weeks Or Less

CONTENT :

Part I: Background to the menopause

Introduction

If you don't like something change it; if you can't change it, change the way you think about it.
- Mary Engelbreit

This quote I find is particularly appropriate to menopause; we cannot change what happens naturally to our bodies, as is the case when menopause starts, however we can change the way we *think* about it, and therefore how we manage it for ourselves. In a world where there is constant media attention and social pressure to stay young, with a lot of negativity around aging, it helps to adapt a positive approach and change how we look at aging, which menopause is a natural part of. This allows us to remain healthy and happy, as we progress through this natural stage of life. The menopause is a natural stage of change in every woman's life, and not a stage of decline, if we manage it positively and proactively.

Although I had been working with women for years helping them manage their health issues, I came to write this book when I myself developed the symptoms of menopause, and my real curiosity was raised. When I asked women I was coaching (on other health issues), about their menopause experience, I discovered a lot of women are suffering in silence and don't find it easy to discuss the issues they are experiencing.

Until I raised the subject with them, and they found someone who could relate to their issues, they became really animated and very keen to speak to me about it.

This eBook will show you the best possible ways to manage the common symptoms of menopause naturally, and help you get back in control of your life in 6 weeks or less, so you can live a healthy and happy life while experiencing menopause.

Why I Wrote This Book

I've worked as a nurse and a midwife, and saw first-hand women seeking help to manage their health and more recently their symptoms of menopause. I could see that during menopause, women often suffer from reduced self-confidence and self-esteem, and so often allowed doctors to take control of managing their symptoms for them.

All too often, women were prescribed medications that they didn't necessarily want but put trust in their doctor saying, 'The Doctor knows best!'

I also spent some years marketing for some of the world's largest pharmaceutical companies, and know first-hand how data can be used to convince doctors that their prescription products are the best option for their patients.

The truth is *no one knows you better than you know yourself*. Recognizing this prompted me to train as a health coach to empower women going through perimenopause to make informed decisions for themselves regarding their own health management. When it comes to looking after our health, there are so many alternatives to prescription drugs out there, with multiple health benefits to be gained, and without the harmful side effects.

The bottom line is: <u>It's your body, your life and your choice</u>. When you're fully informed and aware of the various options open to you, you can make an informed decision as to what's the best treatment option for you. When I first started to experience the symptoms of menopause, it promoted me to find out more. So many of the resources I came across recommended the easy, yet dangerous pharmaceutical options of HRT or anti-depressants. I'm not a doctor or scientist, I am a Nurse, a midwife, and a health coach, but most importantly I'm going through and experiencing menopause first-hand. I have spoken with many women and menopause experts, so I'd like to share the insights I've gained and give you the keys to freedom from menopause.

Chapter 1

What is Menopause?

Menopause is the term used to signify the end of menstruation in women. It is when a woman stops ovulating and therefore stops having periods. It marks the end of the childbearing phase of a women's life. The term 'Menopause' has gained much negativity and is suggestive of a great deal more than the basic fact. The reason why menopause is the cause of anxiety and fear amongst women is due to the significant changes in hormones which occur and the enormous negative impact it can have on our bodies.

Aging is a process that is intrinsically linked with menopause. As we gain in years, our bodies' age and menopause naturally happens as part of that process. Every woman goes through this phase, however the symptoms they experience and how they manage and cope with their menopause varies considerably. While there is no 'one size fits all' approach, there are many things we can do that will help us through this time of huge transition leading to minimal disruption and discomfort.

For most women, menopause occurs between the age of forty-seven and fifty-three. This is generally considered to be the natural age for menopause, although there are many exceptions.

During menopause many women experience a variety of symptoms; the most common being hot flashes from hormonal imbalances. Some women can have lots of problems during this transitional phase of life, and find they need lots of assistance to treat the symptoms of menopause.

Whether the onset of menopause occurs early or late for you can be influenced by many factors, such as:

- How many follicles (egg sacs) you were born with and the rate at which they deteriorate play a role.
- Life style factors – heavy smokers, long-term smokers, or current smokers reach menopause earlier than average.
- Women treated for a variety of illness, such as depression, epilepsy, or some childhood cancers, also reach menopause earlier than average.

6

- Women who have used supplemental Estrogen such as the contraceptive pill or hormone treatment for In Vitro Fertilization (IVF) during the previous 5 years tend to experience menopause later.
- Women who have been pregnant more than once may start menopause slightly later, while those who've never been pregnant, may have an earlier menopause.

The Stages of Menopause

Let's take a look at the various stages of menopause and the symptoms associated with each stage. The word menopause is broadly used to describe a whole raft of changes going on in the body before, during and after that actual starting point.

Here is a description of different stages of menopause to be aware of:

Premature Menopause

Menopause is a natural event that occurs in every woman's life. It is an indicator of the end of a woman's reproductive years. In some cases, women may experience early menopause, and this is commonly referred to as premature menopause.

Premature menopause happens when a woman stops menstruating before her natural age to do so. If it occurs for women in their twenties or thirties, this is considered premature menopause.

The causes of premature menopause vary widely. It will occur in any condition where the ovaries can no longer function; for instance, if radiation is applied to the ovaries, or if the ovaries have been surgically removed due to disease.

Climacteric

This is a term used to denote gradual physical changes in the body due to naturally lowered production of hormones as the ovaries run out of eggs; usually this happens during our forties. There are numerous gradual changes which mark the process of menopause. Like puberty, it does not happen suddenly. The body shows many signs that menopause is nearing.

Pre-menopause

This is the 'child bearing' stage in a women's life prior to any signs of the menopause appearing. Often described as the time in a women's life from the onset

8

of her 1st menstruation to the last, this usually occurs in her late 40's or early fifties.

Peri-menopause

Peri-menopause is the phase leading up to menopause, and usually includes the 12 months after the last period, when the production of female hormones go into decline. The word 'peri' means 'around'. For some the peri-menopause can last 3-15 years but averages between 3-6 years. During the initial peri-menopause phase, women begin to notice the signs of changes in hormone levels, while continuing to ovulate and menstruate. These include:

- Irregular periods
- The onset of hot flashes
- Marked mood swings can also be common during this phase

During Peri-menopause, women are often still fertile and can become pregnant. However, the indicators are there to tell you that you are approaching menopause, and there are fewer chances of getting pregnant. This phase is marked by a considerable rise in the level of your Follicle Stimulating Hormones (FSH),the hormone that encourages the ovary to produce the ovum (or egg).

9

Post-menopause

The term 'Post-menopause' is used to denote the phase of a women's life after menopause. Once a woman has gone 12 months without a menstrual cycle occurring, she has reached full menopause, and is now in the post-menopause period of her life. The ovaries at this time no longer release eggs, produce much less Progesterone and Estrogen and pregnancy is no longer possible.

Hormone Havoc!

What's happening in the transition from the regular menstrual cycle to menopause?

Some women sail through menopause with minimal disruption to their lives, while some experience varying degrees of distress. Some symptoms occur incessantly during menopause and so we try to learn effective ways to treat them. To do this, let's begin by understanding what's going on in the body that causes these changes to take place.

Hormones are chemical messengers, which are released into the blood stream to affect an organ in another part of the body. During the normal menstrual cycle (better known as a period), the pituitary gland in the brain releases what's known as Follicle-Stimulating Hormone (FSH) in the first half of the menstrual cycle, causing levels of Estrogen (also known as the "female hormone") to rise. Estrogen plays an important role in keeping women healthy, especially by helping to build strong bones. Estrogen also makes the lining of the uterus (womb) grow and thicken. This lining of the womb is a place that will nourish the embryo if a pregnancy occurs.

At the same time the lining of the womb is growing, a substance called Lutenising hormone (LH) is released from the pituitary gland in the brain and an egg, or ovum, in one of the ovaries starts to mature. At around day 14 of an average 28-day cycle, the egg leaves the ovary, known as ovulation. At the same time the Corpus Luteum (the part of the ovary remaining after the egg has been released) and the Adrenal Glands also stimulate the production of progesterone.

After the egg has left the ovary, it travels through the Fallopian tube to the Womb. Hormone levels rise and help prepare the wall of the womb for pregnancy. If the egg is not fertilized, hormone levels drop, and the thickened lining of the womb falls away, causing bleeding – better known as the menstrual period.

11

As part of the normal aging process, the ovaries run out of eggs. When eggs are no longer produced, menopause happens, because the ovaries stop producing the hormones Estrogen and Progesterone. As a result of the hormone levels dropping, a woman's menstrual periods stop completely. Aside from controlling fertility, the hormones Estrogen and Progesterone have other functions in the body. When our bodies are out of eggs, (usually in our mid-forties), our hormone levels fluctuate, that is they are high one minute and low the next. With these fluctuations come a variety of symptoms, causing varying degrees of distress for us. Over time the hormone levels start to drop naturally, and then remain consistently low in the 'Post – menopause' stage of life.

By understanding how hormones operate and their effects on the body it helps explain how symptoms develop, and what we can do to influence them in a positive way, thereby reducing the negative effects causing symptoms associated with menopause.

Our bodies are designed to protect us at all times. Our adrenal glands situated above our kidneys produce adrenaline and cortisol (better known as the fight or flight hormones) and release them into the blood stream in times of stress to protect us. It's a primitive function, which was particularly useful when we were hunters and gatherers. However these hormones are less helpful to us in present day, since our lives have become increasingly demanding with daily stressors, such as traffic, raising children, juggling work with home commitments, and constant deadlines to meet.

The raised cortisol levels circulating in the body work on the enzyme 'Aromatase', encouraging our bodies to lay down fat around our waist. The idea being that, when our bodies are ready to fight or flee mode in times of danger, the fat cells are easily accessible by the liver to breakdown into an energy source – glucose.

During peri-menopause, when the ovaries stop producing Estrogen and levels are naturally dropping, our bodies (in protection mode) want to hang onto those fat cells, as they become the primary source of Estrogen production.

The fat gained around the waist becomes another stressor, causing us to release more cortisol into the blood stream, and the vicious cycle continues, making it harder and harder to control the weight gain.

The Functions of Estrogen in the body

The primary function of Estrogen is to develop female secondary sexual characteristics. These include;
- Breasts

- Lining of the womb
- Regulation of the menstrual cycle

It also:

- Plays a major role in fertility and development of the fetus (unborn baby) during pregnancy.
- Slows down height increase in women during puberty, speeds up burning of body fat and reduces muscle bulk.
- Stimulates lubrication of the vagina and thickens the vaginal wall while increasing blood vessels to the skin.
- Increases bone formation.
- Helps with the blood clotting mechanism.
- Increases HDL (good cholesterol) and triglycerides, and decreases LDL (bad cholesterol).
- Causes salt and water retention.
- Reduces bowel motility and increases cholesterol in bile.
- Improves lung function.
- Estrogen is considered to play a very important role in women's mental health – a sudden reduction in the level of Estrogen in the blood correlate with significant lowering of mood.
- Improves collagen content and quality, which keeps elasticity in our skin and other connective

tissues, and improve blood supply to the skin.

Progesterone Stimulates and Regulates Various Functions in the Body

- It helps prepare the body for conception and pregnancy and regulates the monthly menstrual cycle.
- It encourages the growth of milk-producing glands in the breast during pregnancy.
- It plays a key role in maintaining a pregnancy until it's time for delivery.
- It plays a role in sexual desire.
- High progesterone levels are believed to be partly responsible for symptoms of premenstrual syndrome (PMS), such as breast tenderness, feeling bloated and mood swings.
- Progesterone also reduces anxiety and increases sleepiness.
- It helps to build and maintain bones.
- It slows the digestive process.
- It promotes appetite and fat storage.

When we see the huge variety of functions hormones have within the body, it's hardly surprising we develop a wide range of symptoms during and after the menopause - when levels fluctuate, and eventually remain low.

Signs & Symptoms of Menopause

As we age, the ovaries gradually become less responsive to FSH and LH released in the brain. This causes ovulation and menstrual cycles to become irregular, and eventually stop altogether. Several other symptoms may start to show at the same time, including;

- Pre- menstrual syndrome (PMS) may worsen initially with:
  - Abdominal cramps
  - Sleep disturbances
  - Anxiety with no apparent cause
  - Inability to concentrate
  - Forgetfulness
  - Bleeding more or less than previously
  - Lower sex drive

- Short-term unpredictable flashes, with sweating and sometimes palpitations, causing discomfort and disturbance of the normal sleep pattern.
- Symptoms of the urinary and vaginal area - shrinkage of the sex organs, with less vaginal lubrication and urinary issues.
- Shrinkage of breasts.

- Weight gain.
- Underarm and pubic hair becomes sparse.
- Episodes of uncharacteristic behavior e.g. irritability or mood changes.
- Gradual thinning of the skin.
- Loss of bone mass, possibly leading to osteoporosis.
- Slow increase in blood cholesterol levels that increase our risk of heart disease.

During peri-menopause (before actual menopause occurs), symptoms generally occur because of irregular fluctuations in hormone levels. After menopause, symptoms decline because Estrogen and Progesterone levels remain consistently low.

Premenstrual syndrome (PMS)

It is extremely common in the time approaching menopause to experience irregular periods, and worsening of PMS. This is when the body's reserve of eggs to be fertilized runs out, and before there is a reduction of follicle stimulating hormone (FSH) and Lutenising hormone (LH). When there is no egg being produced, the levels of Progesterone remain low, and therefore there is no trigger for a period to flow, prolonging the time between periods from the regular 28-day cycle to a period possibly every 8 – 10 weeks.

17

During this time the symptoms of PMS may worsen with:

- Increased levels of fluid retention
- Bloating
- Abdominal cramps
- Anxiety
- Mood swings
- Sleep disturbances
- Some women experience a shortening of their cycle while in some the signs of menopause are a lengthening of the cycle
- Some women experience very heavy flow, for others the flow is decreased.

Hot Flashes (Tropical moments!)

When it comes to menopause, the most common symptom known and experienced by women would appear to be hot flashes. The time period during which the average woman experiences hot flashes ranges from one to five years. Women, who have had their ovaries surgically removed often experience more severe symptoms. Hot flashes can occur at any time of the day or night. If you wake up to find yourself soaked in sweat, it can be an indicator that you have had a hot flash in your sleep.

Hot flashes are short-term, unpredictable widening of

blood vessels with a sudden increase in your body temperature; flashing of the head, face and neck area accompanied by profuse sweating; sometimes palpitations (feeling of your heart pounding in your chest) causing huge discomfort.

The effects of the hot flash can last from less than one minute to up to five minutes, and can happen as frequently as five episodes in the space of an hour.

There has been a considerable amount of research carried out to try to discover the cause of hot flashes, without any real conclusive findings. It has been established that there is some correlation between lower Estrogen levels in the body, and a reduction in the sweating and shivering thresholds (known as the thermo-neutral zone in the brain). Although the mechanism through which this occurs is not yet known.

Weight Gain

Of all the menopausal symptoms women endure; gaining weight may be the cruelest blow of all. It's not good for our confidence or self-esteem, and because the weight tends to gather around our waist, it can lead to other health problems as well, making us more susceptible to heart disease, Type 2 Diabetes and even some cancers.

A large percentage of women put on weight as they go through menopause, and the average gain is 12 to 15 pounds—the so-called 'middle age spread'. Hormone imbalances play a big role in the ability to control weight. Along with the effect of raised cortisol levels on weight control mentioned earlier, growing older contributes to weight gain because our metabolism slows, meaning we don't burn calories as fast as when we were younger. Also, due to lifestyle changes and possible health issues, we may not be as active as we previously were. Changes in hormones, a natural tendency towards reduced muscle mass, lifestyle, and genetic factors all come into play.

Gaining weight at any age is not a matter of will power or simple Maths. If you take in more calories than you use, you store the extra calories as fat and you gain weight. If it was as simple as reducing your calorie intake, we wouldn't have any weight issues, it's a lot more complicated than that. Then add in menopause and the natural aging process, and balance becomes much harder to control.

The loss of Estrogen makes weight control difficult as our bodies rely on fat cells for Estrogen production. So our body works to convert calories into fat to increase Estrogen levels—and fat cells are much less efficient at burning calories compared with muscle cells. A decrease in Progesterone causes water retention and bloating, much like the bloating that is felt prior to, or during the menstrual period.

You can reduce your chances of gaining extra pounds and even lose what you've gained if you follow my guidelines in this book.

Episodes of Uncharacteristic Behavior - Irritability or Mood Changes

Reduced Estrogen levels also cause:

- Mood changes - Estrogen influences the amount of serotonin (a substance in the body, called a neurotransmitter, which primarily works on our brain and mood) produced in the body.
- Poor memory and attention span.
- Reduced ability to concentrate.

Stress can be the culprit behind additional imbalances in hormones and neurotransmitters that affect mood. Stress negatively impacts our mental function, thyroid function, digestive function and especially blood sugar imbalances. Stress has also been linked to the menopausal symptoms: hot flashes and low libido.

21

Insomnia

Insomnia during the peri-menopause phase is mainly due to frequent night sweats, which may lead to sleep disorders. Mood swings and depression may also lead to sleep problems. However, it is important to ensure you get sufficient sleep. Inadequate sleep often leads to many health problems, such as weight gain and irritability. I'll elaborate on this more in Key No. 4.

Genitourinary Syndrome of Menopause (GSM)

The genitourinary signs and symptoms of menopause are better known as symptoms in the bladder and vaginal area, as well as the opening to the bladder (known as the urethra). The symptoms are yet again due to decreasing levels of Estrogen and other steroid hormones. They can include:

- Burning and irritation of the vaginal area, or entry to the bladder.
- Dryness, discomfort, or pain with intercourse.
- Problems passing urine – needing to go to the toilet in a hurry (urinary urgency), or needing to pass urine more frequently (urinary frequency).
- Pain, such as burning or stinging sensation when trying to pass urine (medically know as dysuria).
- Recurrent urinary tract or vaginal infections.

- An increase in severity of stress incontinence (leaking of urine when coughing, laughing or exercising).

Most of the bladder or vaginal symptoms occur due to reduced Estrogen levels, which cause reduced collagen and elastin (substances which add elasticity and firmness to the walls of these organs). A lack of these substances cause thinning of the walls of the vagina and urethra, altered function of muscles in the region, loss of elasticity and flexibility and diminished blood supply.

These changes increase our chance of contracting vaginal infections. I recommend monitoring for signs and symptoms of vaginal infections, such as an itchy feeling in your vagina, sometimes coupled with a burning sensation. This is also a time when you will find it somewhat difficult to indulge in sexual intercourse. Intercourse might become something that causes discomfort and pain in your vaginal area.

GSM affects about half of all postmenopausal women, but surveys show that women are hesitant to discuss these symptoms with their healthcare providers, and vice versa.

Shrinkage of breasts

During the peri-menopause, as the levels of Estrogen, Progesterone, and *Prolactin begin to fluctuate, your breasts may feel tender and more lumpy. Breast discomfort during the peri-menopausal years is usually cyclical—than means around the time of your period you may feel these symptoms more and then notice that they decrease a few days into your period. Feelings of Fullness may also occur.

At menopause, your hormone levels continue to drop, resulting in breast tissue that's less dense and fattier. You'll also notice physical changes in your breasts. Estrogen keeps the connective tissue of your breasts hydrated and elastic. In the absence of Estrogen, the breasts shrink because the ducts and mammary glands shrink, and the breasts become less firm and lose their shape.

*Prolactin is a hormone produced in the pituitary gland, in the brain, named because of its role in lactation (milk production). It also has other wide-ranging functions in the body from acting on the womb and ovaries, to influencing and regulating the immune system.

Depression

According to Dr. Stacey Gramann, leading Psychiatrist in the UK, each year in the United States 1.3 million women reach menopause. An estimated 20% of these women experience depression. A personal or family history of major depression, postpartum depression, or depressive episodes experienced with periods, seem to be major risk factors for developing depression in the peri-menopausal period.

However, Peri-menopausal Depressive Syndrome is a risk even in women without a history of depression. Depression is approximately twice as common in women as in men (21% vs 12.7%). Moreover, depressive episodes are recorded as recurring more often, for longer periods and symptoms appear to be more profound and impairing for women than for men.

Hypothyroidism is an independent risk factor for depression, which can occur as we age, and may require monitoring as we age. Anemia is another physiological issue, which may arise with peri-menopause, can also lead to depressive episodes.

Other tell-tail signs of menopause include physical changes such as; wrinkles, thinning of hair or the onset of skin problems like acne.

Symptoms tend to last or get worse the first year or more after menopause. Over time, hormone levels peter out to low levels, and many symptoms improve or go away. To what degree we experience symptoms of menopause depends on how we best manage the natural reduction in hormone levels. Therefore to minimize the uncomfortable symptoms, I hope to show you how to balance your hormones naturally, so that you can enjoy this time of your life, and look forward to many more years of health and happiness.

Why naturally?
You don't need to add the worry and risk of ingesting synthetic substances into your bodies at a time that you're struggling to maintain good health as it is.

Chapter 2

What's the Deal with HRT or Hormone Replacement Therapy?

For so many women the world over that experience menopausal symptoms, we have to make a decision whether or not to go down the route of taking hormone replacement therapy (HRT) to relieve our debilitating symptoms, and to protect ourselves from developing other chronic diseases.

For some this decision is easy and for them HRT is not an option, especially if they have:

- A family history of Estrogen sensitive cancers such as:
  - Breast
  - Uterine (womb)
  - Ovarian
  - Endometrial (lining of the womb)
- High blood pressure (Hypertension)
- Heart disease

- History of clotting disorders

HRT is not an option for these as women, as there is well documented evidence of increased risk of developing breast cancer and or an abnormal mammography, heart disease, venous thromboembolic events (VTE), blood clotting disorders, strokes and gallbladder disease. As well as, there is an increased risk of developing Estrogen sensitive cancers.

For lots of women who don't consider themselves in the 'at risk' group, they find themselves reading lots of information and wading through research to make the decision of whether or not to take HRT, or find alternative therapies to relieve their disruptive symptoms.

Over the last 5 to 6 decades, there has been a lot of debate and controversy relating to HRT, primarily due to the conflicting findings from the vast array of clinical trials conducted on various different HRT's.

The first HRT preparations became available to women back in the 1940s, and over the following 20 years increased in popularity, reaching a peak by the 1960s. It revolutionized the management of the menopause, with HRT being prescribed quite frequently to menopausal women for the relief of their most disturbing symptoms; such as hot flashes, night sweats, sleep disturbances, mood swings and further issues, such as urinary frequency and vaginal dryness. It was especially prescribed for its perceived benefit in the prevention of Osteoporosis.

Two large studies of HRT and their use to treat the menopause were undertaken in the 1990's. The Women's Health Initiative (WHI), a randomized clinical trial, was conducted in the US, whilst the "Million Women Study" (MWS), was an observational questionnaire study conducted in the UK.

Both studies published in 2002 and 2003 respectively, raised huge concerns around the safe use of HRT in women. The main safety concerns related to an increased risk of being diagnosed with breast cancer, and that the use of HRT seemed to increase the risk of heart disease.

Within the WHI, there were two study groups: one cohort of women was taking Estrogen alone, and was compared with *placebo; the other cohort of women was taking different forms of HRT containing both Estrogen and Progesterone, also compared to a *placebo group.

A placebo is a simulated or otherwise medically ineffectual treatment for a medical condition intended to deceive the recipient, i.e. a dummy pill.

The test group, given the combination of Estrogen and Progesterone, had a 29% higher rate of coronary heart disease compared to the placebo group. The same group had a 41% increase in the rate of strokes; twice the number of blood clots; a 26 percent increase in invasive breast cancer rates and the rate of cardiovascular disease increased by 22%.

Women in the Estrogen-alone study were more likely to have heart disease risk factors such as high blood pressure, high blood cholesterol, diabetes and obesity. They also showed higher rates of breast cancer diagnoses, according to the research findings published in the Journal of American Medical Association (JAMA) in 2002.

Following publication of the findings in 2002, when the study was stopped prematurely due to the safety concerns raised, there was a marked reduction in the prescribing of HRT's. Approximately 12 months later, a substantial drop in the incidence of breast cancer was recorded in the USA. Several other countries (UK, Canada, Australia, Belgium and France, to mention just a few) subsequently reported similar decreases.

The "Million Women Study" published findings in 2003, and found the use of HRT by women aged 50-64 years in the United Kingdom over the past decade has resulted in an estimated 20,000 extra breast cancer cases, 15,000 associated with Estrogen and Progesterone treatments (Lancet 2003; 362: 419-427).

Later findings from the 2 studies mentioned above show lower incidence of breast cancer risk in women after five years.

A follow up study to the Women's Health Initiative was published in The Journal of the American Medical Association (JAMA) in 2003. This suggested that the relatively short-term combined Estrogen plus Progesterone use increased the incidence of breast cancer, which were diagnosed at a more advanced stage compared with placebo. They also found substantial increases in the percentage of women with abnormal mammograms*. Their results suggest HRT containing Estrogen and Progesterone may stimulate breast cancer growth and hinder breast cancer diagnosis (JAMA 2003; 289: 3243-3253).

Mammogram – a test done to check the breast for lumps and/or breast cancer.

31

HRT & the Increased Risk of Breast Cancer

In a cumulative analysis published in The Lancet of 51 studies on the incidence of breast cancer in Women who took HRT compared to women who never took HRT, the analysis demonstrated the risk of having breast cancer diagnosed increased in women taking HRT. The risk also increased with increasing duration of HRT use. The analysis also showed the effect is reduced after stopping HRT.

Reference – Breast cancer and HRT: Collaborative reanalysis of data from 51 epidemiological studies of 52,705 women with breast cancer, and 108,411 women without breast cancer. The Lancet; Oct 11, 1997; 305-9084; Academic Research Library

HRT & the Increased Risk of Blood Clots

HRT for the management of menopausal symptoms and related disorders is associated with an increased risk of venous thromboembolism (blood clots). The increased risk is twofold to fivefold for women taking HRT. Similarly, there is evidence that by comparison, synthetically produced Progesterone's increase the risk of venous thromboembolism. The use of Estrogen alone has been associated with a 1.2–1.5-fold increased risk compared with those who never used HRT. The relative risk of developing blood clots in women who take HRT seems to be even greater if the women have preexisting risk factors for developing blood clots, such as obesity, immobilization and fractures (broken bones).

Reference - The American College of Obstetricians and Gynecologists: WOMEN'S HEALTH CARE PHYSICIANS COMMITTEE OPINION. Number 556; April 2013.

In 'The Heart and Estrogen/Progestin Replacement Study' (HERS) trial, the rate of venous thromboembolic events was increased nearly 3-fold in the HRT group compared with placebo. Risk for blood clots was increased 5-fold in the first 90 days following a heart attack.

HRT & the Increased Risk of Stroke

According to clinical studies on women taking HRT who had a history of cerebrovascular disease (stroke), the HRT did not prevent them from developing another stroke, or death. In fact their risk increased and the neurological impairment was greater, having had a stroke.

HRT & the Increased Risk of Gall Bladder Disease

The gallbladder is situated in the abdomen and is used to store bile produced by the liver and release it into the digestive system to help digest the food we eat.

Gallbladder disease includes the development of stones produced from bile salts, which cause inflammation of the gallbladder and is associated with severe pain; necessitating surgical removal. Research conducted as part of the Million Women Study involved more than 1.3million women aged 50 to 69, and found that women who take HRT tablets almost double their risk of developing gall bladder disease. It found the chances of having the gall bladder removed surgically were increased slightly by using HRT patches or gels, but taking the treatment in pill format raised the risk twofold.

Natural Progesterone Cream – Creating an Unhealthy Balance!

There was the perception that if Estrogen causes a lot of the health risks associated with HRT, and Progesterone counteracts or balances the effects of Estrogen in the body, then it makes sense that increasing progesterone levels should help with symptom relief.

Dr. John Lee took this simplistic idea and produced and promoted 'Natural Progesterone Cream' as the newest and safest treatment for menopause on the market.

The term 'Estrogen dominance' was used to describe the relative increase in the amount of Estrogen that our bodies are exposed to from prescriptions, hormone treated animal products and Xenoestrogens in our environment (discussed later). The theory was that by taking a 'natural progesterone cream' it would counter balance the effects of Estrogen dominance and reduce the symptoms associated with it.

However what actually happened was very different. Progesterone cream dissolves in fat and can be stored in fatty tissue. The levels of Progesterone steadily increase within fat tissue with prolonged use; after some time the amount being released through the application of cream to the skin, along with the Progesterone being released from the fatty tissues, cause levels to be consistently elevated in the body.

Our bodies have the ability to convert the extra Progesterone into either testosterone (the male hormone) or Estrogen leading to even greater levels of both these hormones circulating. This compounds 'Estrogen dominance', instead of alleviating it as was the intention of taking the progesterone in the first place. Therefore the body is thrown into a dangerous hormone imbalance that does not promote good health. Dr. John Lee has agreed since that taking progesterone in any form over the long term is not good medicine, and not a good balance.

Bioidentical Hormones - Not a Healthy Alternative

'Bioidentical' refers to hormones that are not produced in the body, but are produced in the lab and are similar to our own hormones from the biochemical perspective. The idea is that we can have hormones produced in the lab or pharmacy which are tailored to our individual hormone needs. Bioidentical hormones include Estrone, Estradiol, Estriol, Progesterone, Testosterone, Dehydroepiandrosterone (DHEA) and cortisol, all of which are naturally produced in our bodies. Since our own bodies produce these, it is perceived that we are only taking substances that naturally occur in the body anyway, so what's the harm in that?

The bottom line is that although they are often called 'natural', they are still synthetic chemicals produced in a lab or pharmacy to mimic our own hormones, and are unnatural, ineffective and dangerous.

Dr. Marlyn Glenville, leading expert in nutritional health for women, would not recommend bio-identical hormone therapy for a number of reasons:

1. By supplementing the body with hormones, which naturally decrease during peri-menopause, we are going against nature by trying to boost the levels instead of helping to

body to adjust to our new fluctuating and lowering hormone levels.

2. Sooner than later we will need to stop taking the hormones so really we are just delaying the process of helping our bodies adjust to the lower hormone levels.

3. These are still synthetic substances we are putting into our bodies, and are not necessarily prescription. Therefore women can access them without medical supervision, which could wreak havoc on their bodies.

There is a perceived belief that this type of HRT is safer than conventional prescription-only HRT, because it is tailored to the individual, but there are no randomized trials to show this. There have been a number of women in Australia who have been diagnosed with womb cancer, who were taking Bioidentical hormone therapy.

Don't let celebrities influence you, or let the media pull the wool over your eyes – *they are not natural products, they are drugs, and they are not licensed.*

HRT products (pills, pessaries, gels or patches), alongside their increased risk of causing major health concerns, are not without their relatively minor side effects – bloating, breast tenderness, break through bleeding, nausea and headaches. So while possibly relieving some symptoms, they can be causing others.

While Estrogen-only or Estrogen & Progesterone HRT's might seem like an effective way of managing hot flashes and thinning bones, they have annoying side effects with worrying risks, and huge health concerns.

When we have healthy alternatives which offer additional health benefits, personally I feel it's a no-brainer - why would we put our lives at risk?

Part II:

6 Keys To Unlock And Free Yourself From Menopause Naturally

Chapter 3

No 1: The Food We Eat

Now that we know what's going on in our bodies when Menopause occurs, and the effects of hormone replacement therapy (HRT), doesn't it make more sense to look at the alternatives? I'm not suggesting for a moment that we just shut up and put up with symptoms. Life is too short to have to put up with the intolerable symptoms of Menopause! There are other ways to keep our bodies in optimum health, while at the same time managing symptoms effectively. The way I see Menopause is that our bodies have been locked into this unhealthy position, and with the right keys, we can unlock the codes and free ourselves from Menopause, opening the gates to optimum health.

In the next 6 chapters I will outline the 6 keys which unlock the codes to your freedom from Menopause.

Each key unlocks a code, which will give you partial freedom, but when you use all the keys together, as recommended, then you get complete freedom; so you can enjoy great health – the true wealth.

Can the food you eat really help with menopausal symptoms?

The answer is a resounding *YES*. The saying 'You are what you eat' rings true. Never is it more evident than when I see a client of mine implement the changes I recommend to their eating habits, to discover it has a hugely positive effect on their menopausal symptoms.

Phytoestrogens

Phytoestrogens (Phyto means plant) are naturally occurring chemicals found in plants which are thought to mimic the actions of Estrogen in the body, but at a much more subtle level. There are 3 different types of Phytoestrogens; *Isoflavones, Lignans* and *Coumestans.*

Isoflavones are of particular importance when going through the menopause, as they are known to compete with Estrogen for the same receptor sites, thereby decreasing the health risks of excess Estrogen. If during menopause the body's natural levels of Estrogen drops,

Isoflavones can compensate this by binding to the same receptor, thereby easing menopause symptoms as a result.

The best way to get Isoflavones is in the form of soya or soya-based foods. The highest amounts of soy Isoflavones can be found in soy nuts and tempeh, while lesser amounts are in Soya milk, yogurt and bread. Soy comes in many forms, so you have lots of choices for adding soy Isoflavones to your diet. It's also considered that soybeans in their whole food form (versus soy protein alone), are a healthier form. Much like most other foods, the closer they are to their natural form, the more beneficial they are to us from a nutritional and menopausal perspective.

Isoflavones are short-acting. So when using soy for health reasons, try to eat it throughout the day, rather than all at once. Aim to eat 40 mg - 80 mg of Isoflavones each day. In addition to soy foods, Isoflavones are found in high amounts in chickpeas and lentils.

Linseed or Flaxseeds are the richest food source of the *Lignans*. Research suggests they may have just enough of an Estrogen effect to put a dampener on the uncomfortable symptoms of menopause. Lignans are found in rye, oats, barley and wheat germ and in the vegetables broccoli and carrots.

Coumestans is the third type of Phytoestrogen. Food sources high in Coumestans include split peas, pinto beans, lima beans and specially alfalfa and clover sprouts.

Again, as a phytoestrogen, Coumestans imitate the effect of Estrogen, so the body reacts as if it's Estrogen, just in a milder form. Therefore it reduces the harmful effect of high levels of Estrogen, while tricking to body into thinking it has Estrogen, so reducing the symptoms of menopause.

Xeno-Estrogens

Xeno-Estrogens are manufactured chemical compounds which are a sub group of chemicals known as endocrine disruptors. Xeno-Estrogens specifically mimic the effect of Estrogen in the human body. They are found in our everyday environment and tend to remain under our radar, as some perceive them to be harmless. Unlike Phytoestrogens (natural plant based 'adaptogens' that influence our Estrogen levels in a positive way), Xeno-Oestrogens disrupt the hormone balance in our bodies and mimic the effects of Oestrogen, often boosting levels causing Estrogen dominance. This is particularly

44

harmful when their effect is exerted on hormone-sensitive sites, which may include hormone sensitive tumor cells. This may promote tumor growth of some Estrogen sensitive cancers such as breast or uterine cancer.

Xeno-Estrogens are found in plastics, some detergents, pesticides and herbicides. Xeno-Estrogens also include the residues in the breakdown of pharmaceutically manufactured hormones, such as the contraceptive pill and hormone replacement therapies, which find their way back into our water supply.

To cut down on your exposure to Xeno-Estrogens, where possible:

- Drink bottled water, preferably from glass bottles, as the plastic contained in disposable water bottles sold commercially are also known to contain Xeno-Estrogens.
- Buy organic food such as meat, dairy, fruit and vegetables. If this is not feasible peel all fruit and vegetables prior to use or consumption.
- Keep your use of cling film and/or plastic containers to a minimum and choose to store food in glass or ceramic containers instead.

- Remove food bought in plastic trays from the packaging for storage.
- Buy meats and dairy products which are hormone-free to avoid hormones and pesticides.

Sugar

One of the biggest culprits in our diet for worsening our menopausal symptoms is SUGAR. Sugar, or more appropriately put, refined carbohydrates (white bread, white rice, pastries, biscuits, cake, chocolate bars, soft drinks etc.) play havoc with our hormones. They worsen all symptoms associated with menopause, especially hot flashes, mood swings and our anxiety levels. You don't have to be a diabetic for sugar to cause problems with your health.

How can this be?
When you eat a refined carbohydrate, your blood sugar raises really quickly. Your brain then signals your body to produce extra insulin (the hormone that controls our blood sugars). Insulin helps take sugar out of the bloodstream, usually by converting the excess sugar into fat and storing it in your body.

The more refined carbohydrates you eat, the bigger the increase in insulin levels, the more fat you store and the bigger the drop in your blood sugar levels, leaving you feeling tired and sluggish. This is medically called 'hypoglycemia'. Low blood sugar levels stimulate our adrenal glands to produce the hormones adrenaline and cortisol, better known as the 'stress hormones' (the same hormones we release when we're under pressure or stress). These hormones help the body to release the sugar stores within the body in an effort to correct the low blood sugar levels. At the same time as these hormones are released, our bodies also experience sugar cravings, prompting us to reach for a sugar fix.

We satisfy the craving by eating a carbohydrate snack, which gives us that energy rush (sugar high) followed by feeling tired with food cravings (sugar low). The more sugar or refined carbohydrates we eat, the more we feel the roller coaster ride of sugar highs and lows, causing us to crave refined carbohydrates, fueling the sugar addiction. Using the word sugar can be misleading as white bread, white pasta and white rice are all refined carbohydrates, which don't necessarily taste sweet, yet they cause our blood sugars to soar, having a similar effect as the chocolate bars or fizzy drinks.

With raised sugar levels, our insulin levels rise, which in turn increases the production of testosterone, this is then converted into Estrogen by fat cells in our body, especially around our stomach area. This leads to fluctuating levels of Estrogen and the dreaded symptoms like irritability, anxiety and insomnia all worsen. As we reach menopause, with already fluctuating levels of Estrogen, symptoms can become more intense and can include hot flashes and night sweats as well.

The sequence of events taking place in the body as described above is better known as *Estrogen Dominance*. Besides the natural hormonal fluctuations of menopause, certain lifestyle choices and conditions also contribute to *Estrogen Dominance Syndrome*, especially eating a low-fiber diet, overloading the liver with toxins obtained through the food we eat or from the environment.

Consistently raised sugar levels over a long period of time through eating refined carbohydrates is significant, as it causes sustained excess insulin secretion and can result in various ill health effects such as fatigue, weight gain leading to obesity and eventually, *Type 2 Diabetes*.

So to dramatically improve your symptoms of Menopause, reduce your intake of refined carbohydrates. Instead, try swapping to complex carbohydrates such as wholegrain bread, pasta and brown rice, as well as lots of fruit and vegetables.

For a list of refined carbohydrates see page…

GOOD Fat & BAD Fat

There are many different types of fats we can eat, and they can be divided into lots of categories, but the 2 main groups are:

- Essential (polyunsaturated fats – nuts, seeds, seed oils and oily fish)
- Nonessential (saturated fats – butter, cheese, milk, pastries, cakes etc.).

Saturated fats can only be used by the body for energy, or stored as fat for energy use at a later date. Polyunsaturated fats on the other hand, are used by the body for lots of different functions, most importantly during menopause for balancing hormones, boosting our immunity and to give us healthy skin.

Omega 3, a fatty acid found in polyunsaturated fats, helps the body to produce a hormone called prostaglandin. This helps the body to control metabolism (the rate which we burn calories), and fat burning capacity. Omega 3 also helps the complex carbohydrates mentioned in the last section to control food cravings, burn fat and lose or maintain a healthy weight.

Omega 6 is another fatty acid found in polyunsaturated fats, particularly in nuts seeds such as sunflower, sesame seeds and legumes. Omega 6 can have similarly good effects on the body, but can be harmful if you have low levels of Omega 3. If you are already experiencing variations in your insulin levels caused by the refined carbohydrates you are eating (you'll know if you're having food cravings alternating with bouts of tiredness), Omega 6 can worsen the effects of the high insulin levels and cause inflammation in your body, in the form of joint or muscle pains.

Therefore it's recommended for women going through menopause to boost your intake of Omega 3, specifically to boost the anti-inflammatory effect on the body. During menopause, the amount of Estrogen in a woman's body declines. As Estrogen helps control unhealthy cholesterol, this change can increase the risk of heart disease. Reducing your intake of saturated fats and increasing your intake of polyunsaturated fats, in particular Omega 3, can help you fight heart disease.

For most people, their metabolism slows steadily after age 40. Although we can't control our age, gender or genetics, there are other ways to improve our metabolism. The biggest mistake people make is cutting out fats. It's important to eat good fats (AKA essential fats), such as avocado, olive oil, nuts and oily fish like salmon. While cutting down or out the bad fats (non-essential fats) found in dairy products and processed foods.

For a list of polyunsaturated and saturated fats see page…

Fruit & Vegetables

As you know, the Menopause can be a period of great change and transition in our lives. It helps to be aware of the best fruits and vegetables for menopause relief. It's best to include fruit and vegetables in your diet before, during and after menopause. If you have not yet started to experience any symptoms of menopause, these foods will help your body handle menopause symptoms, if or when they attack. On the other hand, if you've managed to get through menopause, these natural foods will keep you healthy and help your body deal with symptoms that can go on for years. It's never too late to increase your intake of fruit and vegetables to get the health benefits.

How can fruit and vegetables possibly help?
We hear a lot of talk about free radicals these days, but what are they? Are they harmful? Free radicals are substances formed naturally in your body as a by-product of normal functioning. If left to their own devices these free radicals move around our bodies wreaking havoc on other cells, causing damage and leaving you wide open to develop diseases or various health conditions including some cancers.

Our best and most effective line of defense against the damage these free radicals cause is by producing antioxidants. Our best way of getting lots of these antioxidants is not from supplements, but from the food we eat, and in particular fruit and vegetables. As you try to reduce your intake of sugar, or refined carbohydrates, fruit and vegetables are good foods to replace those foods with, so you get double the benefit.

One potentially important antioxidant found in fruits and vegetables is *Boron*. Research suggests that an increased intake of fruit and vegetables rich in antioxidants, including Boron, may improve bone health and reduce the risk of Osteoporosis. This is because Boron improves the absorption of calcium by converting Vitamin D to its active form.

One of the functions of Estrogen is to help lay down calcium to build strong bones. So as the Estrogen levels drop in our body, so too do our calcium levels, which significantly reduces our bone density. This makes us much more susceptible to osteoporosis and breaking bones. Lots of fruits and vegetables are rich sources of calcium. As we progress through menopause, and the Estrogen levels continue to fall, the extra calcium from the extra fruit and vegetables will be put to very good work in maintaining good bone health.

The other great benefit of increasing our fruit and veg intake is that they contain natural plant chemicals known as Phyto-Estrogens. These are very similar in structure to a women's Estrogen. Many experts consider this natural chemical to be beneficial for women who are going through menopause. It may be that it helps relieve menopause symptoms because it provides a similar chemical to the one that is decreasing in your body.

I recommend you eat a wide variety of fresh fruit and vegetables, and include all of the colors of the rainbow to get maximum benefit from them. The different colored fruit and vegetables have varying amounts of different nutrients and antioxidants', so varying your choice means you'll get all the nutrients available. 5 a day absolute minimum!

For a full list of foods containing antioxidants see page ..

Fibre

Not to complicate things too much, but more for clarification, there are 2 forms of fibre: **soluble** and **insoluble**. Both are often contained within the same foods, but they act differently within the body.

Insoluble fibre <u>cannot</u> be digested. It's like the road sweeper passing through your gut, sweeping up the rubbish and waste as it goes, so you can get rid of it. Insoluble fibre keeps your bowels healthy and helps prevent digestive problems, such as constipation, and reduces the risk of developing bowel cancer.

Examples of foods high in insoluble fibre:
- Whole-meal bread

- Wholegrain cereals
- Nuts and seeds

Soluble fibre is different. It <u>can</u> be digested by your body. Soluble fibre has a different role to play. It binds to cholesterol, so that it's less likely to stick to the walls of arteries, causing damage. By eating foods high in soluble fibre it will help get rid of excess cholesterol, lowering your blood cholesterol level helping you stay healthier for longer.

Examples of food high in soluble fibre:
- Oats, barley and rye
- Fruit, such as bananas and apples
- Vegetables, such as carrots, potatoes, peas, beans, lentils and chickpeas
- Golden linseeds (flaxseed)

Fibre is especially beneficial during menopause. As well as sweeping up cholesterol, it also sweeps up old Estrogen, which would otherwise recirculate through the body causing levels to rise, leaving you exposed to the increased risk of breast cancer.

Another benefit to eating a lot of fibre is that it helps control blood sugar levels, keeping them on an even keel. This helps reduce the frequency and severity of hot flashes. As well as this, fibre rich foods create a feeling of satiety and this keeps hunger pangs at bay. Our body uses 10% of its calorie intake for digestion, which increased further by increasing fibre intake. By consuming foods from the plant kingdom, you are feeding the micro-flora in the gut. Recent research has shown that fibre rich foods which contain certain prebiotics affect the expression of certain genes in the gut associated with weight gain and fuel burning in the body.

So when choosing to eat bread, choose high fibre bread, which means it has a minimum of 3 grams of fiber per serving (five or more is even better). In order to have all the benefits of fibre it is important to vary the sources of fibre in your diet. Diets with fruit, vegetables, lentils/beans and whole grains not only provide fibre, but also many other nutrients and food components essential to good health. The digestive system slows down with age, so a high-fibre diet becomes even more important as we get older.

Also make sure you are drinking enough water to help that fibre work through your system. Similar to the effect water has on porridge oats, when you eat fibre and drink water, the water causes the fibre to swell and become sticky, this helps the fibre to work its way through the bowel, binding all the waste products to it. This has a great cleaning effect on the bowel. The more water you drink the more effective the fibre you eat. When enough fluids are not taken in to accompany the fibre, it may cause abdominal discomfort or constipation.

Becoming more aware of the foods you eat, and implementing small changes to your eating habits over weeks, you'll be surprised at the changes you notice in your weight, your mood, your sleep and your overall wellbeing.

Chapter 4

No. Two: Movement is Medicine

I'm sure you've heard and read that exercise is good for you in terms of keeping fit. Now that you're nearing, or are in the throes of peri-menopause, you would probably prefer to slow down and take it easy. However it has been proven that one of the most effective and natural remedies for Menopause is movement or exercise.

Why is this?

Some studies have shown that exercising a few times a week (minimum) can greatly reduce the occurrence of symptoms - including hot flashes - one of the most troublesome symptoms. The benefits of exercise during menopause go far beyond reducing the severity of hot flashes, and can include:

- Effectively reduce stress levels and symptoms of anxiety, irritability or mood changes
- Improve digestion and get the bowels working more efficiently
- Increase energy levels and improve sleep
- Help to manage weight
- Lower risk of heart disease, heart attack and other cardiovascular diseases
- Improve memory and concentration
- Lower risk of osteoporosis
- Improve your overall health

How can exercise do all this?

Effectively reduce stress levels

We mentioned earlier the close link of Cortisol with Estrogen and Progesterone. During menopause, while your body is undergoing hormone changes, the changes can have unexpected effects on the rest of your body, including the nervous and digestive systems.

Drops in Estrogen levels impact other hormones in the body called Cortisol and Adrenaline (stress hormones). When your level of Estrogen is high, Cortisol and Adrenaline are lower, keeping your blood sugar and blood pressure at a healthy level. However, as menopause advances, and the levels of Estrogen are dropping, the levels of Cortisol and Adrenaline can rise.

This constant production of our stress hormones has a direct effect on:

- Our ability to lose weight
- Handle food cravings
- Keep high blood pressure in check
- Keep cholesterol levels down
- Fight off menopausal symptoms; especially hot flashes
- Our ability to sleep
- Digestive issues such as constipation, bloating and indigestion
- Preventing diabetes
- Protection from depression

The difficulty with these stress hormones is that they are designed for fight or flight. Unfortunately in the current environment we can't just 'fight or flight' and therefore use the hormones to our benefit. Instead we have them circulating in our body's causing us stress symptoms such as anxiety, palpitations, nervousness and sleep disturbances. That's where exercise comes in very useful. Through exercise we use up the circulating stress hormones, reducing their levels in the body and bringing about a much calmer, stress-free mind and body, making it easier to work, rest and play! This leaves you with a greater ability to manage menopausal symptoms.

Reduce Digestive Issues

Adrenaline is easily triggered and released when the calming influence of Estrogen is missing. This slows your gut function right down, and when the gut is not working at its optimum level, a range of problems can arise. Food can pass through without being fully broken down causing constipation. At the same time acid can break down the mucous lining of the stomach wall, causing abdominal pain or indigestion associated with gastro-esophageal reflux disease (GERD), peptic ulcer disease, inflammatory bowel disease (IBD), and irritable bowel syndrome (IBS).

Exercise is a very effective means for reducing adrenaline and cortisol levels in the body. With regular movement and exercise, the blood flow improves throughout the body - including your digestive system. Keep your body moving with regular exercise, and you can keep your digestive tract moving too. A consistent exercise routine can help you avoid a sluggish digestive system and ward off the digestive ailments mentioned above.

Increasing Your Energy Levels

If you are experiencing feelings of low energy, fatigue, the need to take a nap, or spend longer in bed, you are not alone. These are very common symptoms of menopause. The primary cause of reduced energy levels in middle-aged women is hormone imbalance. The two hormones Estrogen and Progesterone play a significant role in your sleep cycle, therefore when the levels start to fluctuate and decline, levels of cortisol increase. This has a big impact on your ability to get to sleep, as well as staying asleep, leading to fatigue and low energy.

Estrogen facilitates the deep sleep state (REM Sleep), which helps the body to repair itself and regain energy stores for the following day. With the drop of Estrogen that occurs naturally with age, time spent in restorative (REM) sleep decreases, leaving you feeling constantly drained, with trouble concentrating.

At the same time, Progesterone levels are also decreasing. This hormone stimulates the sleep center, causing feelings of sleepiness, and helps us nod off to sleep at bedtime. In the absence of Progesterone, or with a reduced amount circulating, it can lead to periods of insomnia or sleeplessness, again affecting our energy levels the following day. Many women suffer from an apparent 'brain fog' or inability to concentrate – which researchers attribute to inefficient sleep episodes.

While exercising is the furthest thing from your mind when you're feeling tired and worn out, it's actually the best thing you can do to boost your energy levels. The great benefit of exercise is that it helps the body to produce endorphins - known as the 'Happy Hormone'. Endorphins increase energy levels and reduce symptoms of depression, anxiety and stress naturally, without taking a single pharmaceutical drug. Exercise also cuts down the sleep disturbing night sweats, allowing a better night's sleep, which in turn boosts energy levels during the day. So getting physically active by day leads to better sleep, greater concentration, and reduced 'brain fog'.

Helping to Manage Your Weight

During puberty, the ovaries are producing large quantities of Estrogen and Progesterone. Fat cells also produce Estrogen; however as the body has sufficient levels already from the ovaries, the body is not in need of fat cells, so is not inclined to hold onto them. When Estrogen levels drop, during and after menopause, the opposite happens - the body holds onto fat cells to boost its Estrogen levels. At the same time the metabolic rate slows down (the rate at which the body converts stored energy into working energy), leading to weight gain.

As part of the natural aging process, women after the age of Forty start to lose muscle mass. Some clinical trials are working on the link between lowered Estrogen levels and reduced muscle strength and mass; however the link has not been fully established. Other studies show that a lack of Estrogen may also cause the body to be less efficient at using carbohydrates, including regulation of blood sugars, which increase fat storage and make it harder to lose weight.

Your level of activity is important to counteract what nature is doing to your body. If you're less active and aren't replacing lost muscle mass, your body composition will gradually move towards more fat. Therefore to maintain optimum weight and health it's best to participate in regular exercise, which we will go into greater detail later.

Keeping Your Heart Healthy

During childbearing years, Estrogen helps maintain a healthy heart by increasing good cholesterol (HDL) and triglycerides, while reducing bad cholesterol (LDL) by helping the liver get rid of it through bile in the digestive tract. When approaching menopause, Estrogen levels start to drop and we start losing all of these benefits. At the same time, we may start to gain a few extra pounds, especially around the middle. This combination puts us at a much higher risk of developing heart problems. Fat around the middle (AKA belly fat, visceral fat or central obesity), is known to be much more harmful than the fat we store around our hips and thighs. The belly fat is stored here so that it is close to the liver for easy access in times of need. The problem is the fat that is not required by the liver gets dumped into the blood stream causing problems such as heart disease, high blood pressure and strokes.

Heart disease resulting from menopause can be effectively curtailed through managing stress, healthy eating and plenty of cardiovascular exercise. This can prevent the onset of medical conditions such as high blood pressure, high cholesterol, central obesity, or fatty liver disease.

Exercise as a natural treatment to reduce your risk of heart disease has many benefits to it:

- Increases your good cholesterol (HDL), which, carry's the bad cholesterol to your digestive tract to be disposed of so it can't circulate the body causing you harm.
- Gets you 'heart fit'.
- Reduces stress, which in turn help you control your blood pressure naturally - avoiding the need for medications.
- Helps to maintain muscle mass (including heart muscle), and control weight, reducing the pressure that those extra pounds put on your heart muscles.
- Maintains good blood circulation, which reduces the risk of heart attack, stroke or blood clots.

Lower Your Risk of Osteoporosis

As mentioned previously, Estrogen promotes bone formation by helping to make calcium available to produce good bone strength and density. With the reduction in Estrogen levels, so too may come a reduction in bone mass and bone density. This can lead to a condition known as Osteoporosis (brittle bones) and can leave you at high risk of breaking bones following even the simplest of falls.

Menopause-related bone loss doesn't have to cause you grief, if you take care of yourself, exercise and eat nutritious foods. Menopause in itself does not cause bone loss. Instead, the lack of Estrogen can lead to bone related issues. Not all women in menopause have bone loss. Some women who still have their periods have Osteoporosis, so it is more than likely that your overall health and heredity play a bigger factor than Menopause does on bone loss in women.

Physical activity can slow the process of bone loss after menopause, which significantly lowers your risk of fractures and Osteoporosis. A combination of weight bearing exercises and resistance training are most beneficial to bones during this stage of life. Weight bearing exercises can include walking, running, cycling or aerobics. Resistance or weight training can include using free weights or weighing machines in the gym. Both types of exercise stimulate bones to strengthen because of the association with muscle contraction.

It is important to know that not having enough exercise can greatly increase the risk of Osteoporosis.

Improve Your Overall Health

The benefits of exercise extend far beyond the few I've listed here. Clinical research shows that regular exercise can help reduce your risk for many different diseases and health conditions and improve your overall quality of life. Taking regular exercise and maintaining a healthy weight can help protect you from such issues as:

- Back pain
- Stroke
- Depression
- Anxiety
- Type 2 Diabetes
- Certain cancers

So What Exercise Works Best for Menopause?

The World Health Organization (WHO) recommends all adults up to the age of 64 should do a minimum of 150 minutes of moderate-intensity aerobic physical activity per week, or a minimum of 75 minutes vigorous-intensity aerobic physical activity per week. The aerobic activity should be performed in bouts of at least 10 minutes duration.

The idea of aerobic activity (also known as cardio training), is something that makes use of your large muscle groups while maintaining a raised heart rate and can include: walking running or jogging, cycling, swimming, dancing or aerobic gym classes, to mention just a few.

It's recommended to take a moderate amount of exercise every-day. Beginners start with 10 minutes of light activity, slowly increasing the exercise intensity and duration as it becomes easier. This may seem a huge ask of you if your relatively inactive at the moment, but believe me, by starting with a small amount you'll be amazed at how you're body will get used to it, and then you'll be able to do a little bit more every week. It is difficult at the start, but persevere through the soreness and stiffness, and you'll feel better sooner than later, honestly!

If you already take some exercise, aim to set a goal of 30 – 60 minutes per day most days of the week. If this is not achievable, do as much as you're able to do and build up the amount you do over time. Walking at a moderate pace is always a good start for at least 30 minutes on most days.

Strength training (AKA Resistance training) a couple of times a week is also advisable to help build bone and muscle strength, burn body fat and speed up metabolism. If you are already active and exercising, you may need to increase your level of activity to prevent further weight gain. Examples of strength training include weight machines, dumb bells or kettle bells. You don't have to buy these weights to start with, you could use cans of food or 1kg bags of rice. Start with a level that is heavy enough to tire your muscles in 12 repetitions and progress from there. Other forms of strength training are exercise bands, yoga, Pilates and gardening.

Exercise shouldn't be entirely hard work. Participating in calorie-burning physical activities can be fun as well as good for your body. Varying your workouts can also enhance enjoyment and prevent boredom. If you're not into running on a treadmill, or prefer to be around people when you work out, think about a running, walking or cycling club, the gym or a dance class. Dance can help to build muscle and keep you flexible. With many different styles to choose from; ballroom, jazz, salsa, or Zumba - pick one you think you'll enjoy. Enjoy burning calories and working your muscles, while moving to uplifting music. If you are into gym workouts, machines such as the cross trainer or the stair-master count as cardio workouts too.

Gentle exercise can be beneficial too; especially if your adrenal glands are overworked (adrenal fatigue) and you constantly feel tired. If you're finding it difficult to get your head around having to exercise, why not try Yoga (also a type of strength training) – which has been increasing in popularity over the last decade or so. Often we think of yoga being done by skinny acrobatic-like petite women, but the great thing about Yoga is that you go at your own pace and your own ability. It's not about puffing and panting, but rather pushing your body to do what it will allow you to do, and no further. It's over time, through regular consistent practice that your body gains more movement and flexibility, while at the same time reducing both physical and emotional stress by learning how to relax fully, leading to deeper sleep.

Through studies it has been shown that yoga has been of particular benefit to menopausal women in reducing stress, anxiety and mood swings, while at the same time improving sleep patterns and hot flashes.

Allow yourself four to six weeks to feel the full effects of how a combination of cardio workout and strength training can help you beat the typical menopausal symptoms. Most importantly—do something you enjoy!

Chapter 5

No. 3: Good Hydration

Believe it or not adequate hydration is one of the biggest influencer's in managing your Menopausal symptoms. I cannot emphasize enough the importance of maintaining hydration. Our bodies are made up of at least 2 thirds water and if we neglect our water intake this can cause a whole raft of symptoms.

As you can see from the list below, the symptoms of Menopause are quite similar to symptoms of dehydration. So often when people say they have symptoms of Menopause, it may often be confused with, or worsened by, dehydration. By maintaining adequate hydration on a daily basis, the severity of your Menopausal symptoms can dramatically improve.

Signs of dehydration include:
- Thirst – which can be confused as hunger
- Irritability / inability to concentrate / forgetfulness
- Headache / tension
- Mood swings / anxiety
- Dry and itchy skin
- Bloated stomach / constipation
- Hot Flashes – dehydration can affect the nervous system, which triggers hot flushes. Water is particularly important here because if you sweat a lot with the flushes, that will further dehydrate you, causing a vicious cycle!
- Fatigue / reduced energy levels
- Bladder problems and infections
- Joint pain
- Yellow or amber colored urine – meaning it is too concentrated

There are a variety of factors which influence the amount of water required by the body to maintain hydration, which include; height, weight, gender, how active you are and what other fluids you're drinking. There are lots of ways to calculate how much water you need, but the most common recommendation is to drink between 1.5 – 2 liters (2 ½ - 4 pints) of water per day.

I know lots of people equate drinking lots of **fluids** with drinking lots of **water** but it's not the same thing. Drinking lots of tea, coffee, alcohol or fizzy drinks doesn't count towards hydration. They actually have a diuretic effect, which means they encourage your kidneys to flush water out of your body, *causing further dehydration*!

Water is the best fluid you can drink to rehydrate. It helps the body to detoxify by removing waste products, pollutants and toxins. I know for some people drinking water can be really difficult, as they don't like the taste. If you don't like plain water at all, start by adding one glass of water a day for a few days then slowly increase your intake. You might be surprised at how you develop a taste for it!

If you suddenly start drinking lots of water you may find yourself running to the toilet all day, so increase your intake slowly and this will allow your kidneys and bladder time to adapt.

It's best to start the day with a glass of water as soon as you get up. Having it at room temperature helps to kick-start your metabolism. Chilled water can be harder to digest. If you're not keen on plain water, adding fresh lemon or lime juice to your water can act as a natural flavor enhancer. These fruits are alkalizing to the body; the body works more efficiently in an alkaline state than an acid state. This helps to restore the body's natural PH balance, which is another positive benefit.

Cucumber is another food, which you could add either on its own, with the lemon or lime, or with a few sprigs of mint. All are great healthy additions to water.

I know your probably thinking; *why not just buy flavored waters?* Apart from the expense of that, these commercially packaged waters are not as nutritionally beneficial to you as making up your own fresh.

The Benefits of Drinking Cucumber & Lemon Water

Cucumbers are high in vitamin A and C, and since the vitamins are coming from real food sources and not jars of vitamins, they are much better absorbed and put to good use by the body than if you were to get them from waters marketed as 'containing added vitamins'. Cucumber contains Silica, which is a nutrient particularly good for maintaining healthy bones, good skin, hair and nails, and healthy muscles. It is also high in potassium, which helps to control your blood pressure. Cucumber is rich in antioxidants, which fight off free radicals (produced within the body, but harmful to it) and help the body flush out toxins. This has great anti –aging effects as well as helping you fight diseases. Cucumber also contains lots of vitamin K, which is essential for blood clotting. If cucumber is not your thing, why not try lemon water?

I consider lemons as one of our 'Superfoods'. It has an endless number of benefits; lemons are good sources of vitamin C, which is a water-soluble vitamin and a good antioxidant which helps fight off the free radicals mentioned earlier. One of the other great benefits to lemon water is that it reduces the acidity in the body, and removes uric acid from the joints which causes inflammation.

Drinking little and often is much better for you than trying to knock back big glasses of water all at once. If you keep a glass or bottle of water near you most of the day, and take small sips throughout the day, you'll be surprised at how quickly you'll reach your target intake. Have one last glass of water early evening, that way you won't have to worry about getting up to the toilet in the middle of the night.

Aside from reducing the symptoms of dehydration and Menopause, drinking water has lots of other benefits to it. Water is great for people who are trying to lose weight and cut down on calories. Thirst is often mistaken for hunger causing people to eat, only to cause the body to dehydrate further. When you're hungry, try drinking a glass of water first and wait 15 minutes or so. If you still feel the need to eat after that, you'll know for sure that you're craving food instead of fluids. Water also helps speed up your metabolism so that you burn calories faster. One of the organs responsible for turning fat into energy is the liver, and water helps your liver work more efficiently.

There are certain foods that contain high amounts of water, such as most fruits and vegetables. Eating healthy, non-processed foods like these will not only deal with your hunger, but also add to your water intake for the day. The best part is these foods are also low in calories, so they won't wreck your diet the way fatty snack foods would. Try drinking water 15 to 20 minutes before each meal. This will help you to fill up faster, and therefore eat fewer calories.

80

Stimulant Drinks & The Menopause
Coffee, tea, energy and fizzy drinks

There is a lot of debate around the health effects of coffee, is it good for you or is it bad for you? Depending on which research findings you read, you will see conflicting evidence – some research states it reduces your chances of developing Type 2 diabetes, Alzheimer's and some cancers, while others report the opposite. It's no wonder the jury is out on whether we should drink it or not.

After reading the points on coffee below, there should be no doubt in your mind that you need to kick the habit. The same applies to tea, energy drinks and some fizzy drinks all of which contain varying amounts of caffeine; so when I'm talking about coffee below, I'm including tea, energy drinks and fizzy drinks such as Cola, all of which contain caffeine.

It's widely recommended to cut coffee out completely if you're experiencing certain symptoms associated with menopause, especially:

- Hot flashes
- Irritability
- Poor concentration / memory loss or 'Brain fog'
- Mood swings

- Inability to sleep
- Fatigue

Get rid of it!

Coffee is *pure acid,* and it is a nerve toxin. This acid addiction turns your bloodstream to *sludge.* Coffee is one of the most acidic things you could consume, and does *not* give you energy. It is a virulent nerve toxin that spikes your adrenaline because your body is *fighting to get rid of this poison.* You feel like you're "buzzing" briefly, and then it *robs you* of energy. Do you really think coffee brings your body any nutrition whatsoever?

Caffeine *increases* catecholamine's, your stress hormones. The stress response elicits cortisol and increases insulin. Insulin increases inflammation and this makes you feel lousy, not to mention it increases your risk of mortality related to cardiovascular disease. Caffeine increases relaxation of the muscle that keeps stomach acid from rising into the Esophagus and throat (GERD). The acidity of coffee is associated with digestive discomfort, indigestion, heartburn, and imbalances in your gut flora (also symptoms of menopause). Caffeine also contributes to the surge in hormone levels during menopause, causing hot flashes. Quitting coffee will reduce stimulation of the adrenal glands, and in turn the frequency and severity of hot flashes.

Many women going through menopause complain of digestive symptoms such as heartburn and indigestion. Caffeine also stimulates acid secretion in the stomach; therefore by continuing to drink coffee, or caffeinated drinks, you're helping these digestive symptoms to worsen.

Coffee, filled with milk and sugar, is the epitome of food lacking nutrition density and it makes you feel lousy, too! Coffee drinkers are at risk of having lower levels of serotonin, which is necessary for normal sleep, bowel function, mood and energy levels. That's right - caffeine can disrupt sleep and promote anxiety and depression, symptoms you may have thought were due to your menopause.

Coffee makes you *toxic,* and interferes with the detoxification process of the liver. Coffee is so acidic that it depletes your body of vital minerals such as calcium, magnesium and potassium – your body leaches these alkaline elements from your bones, because it takes 10 parts of alkalinity to eliminate ONE part of acidity from your bloodstream! This is the last thing you need when trying to prevent Osteoporosis and heart disease.

Coffee is totally destructive for your body! The only reason you drink coffee is because you've been conditioned to do so. You take this toxin in every day because of a social hypnosis.

Wake up and quit this toxic addiction!

Cutting caffeine out at the one time you feel you need it to get you through the day can be really difficult. The famous quote from Plato "Necessity is the mother of invention" springs to mind here. If you are finding your menopause symptoms particularly difficult to tolerate and they are getting in the way of you getting on with your life, then in order to start feeling human again, you need to quit your caffeine habit completely. You'll be pleasantly surprised at the results, once you get over the initial withdrawal symptoms.

Similarly to my recommendations to increase your water intake, I recommend reducing your caffeine intake slowly. So if you feel you are a caffeine addict, and the thought of giving it up seems completely impossible, start slowly, by cutting down before cutting out. Set yourself a date in the future, (for example 2 weeks' time) when you can say 'I am now caffeine free'.

Consider keeping the morning caffeine fix initially, while cutting out each of the other cups at 1 to 2 day intervals, starting with the last cup of the day. By doing this you are allowing your cortisol levels to drop in the evening leading to more restful night's sleep. I also recommend you start cutting down on your less busy days (maybe the weekend) so you're not putting yourself under undue pressure. Also, if you are tempted to have a caffeine fix, choose the lower caffeine option. For example if you normally drink strong coffee, try a weaker strength cup, or tea instead. Experiment with caffeine-free teas such as Rooibos or peppermint tea, so that if you're out socializing with friends, you have an alternative to caffeine without really depriving yourself. I personally carry Rooibos tea-bags with me at all times, so that if the caffeine free teas are not available (in a friend's house for instance!) you can ask them for boiled water and add your own caffeine-free tea bag!

Avoiding coffee, tea and energy drinks will require self-discipline initially, but your efforts and persistence will be really worthwhile as you notice your menopause symptoms diminish in frequency and severity after you

85

have quit completely.

If you are a real caffeine addict (as I once was) and the prospect of giving up one of your great pleasures in life fills you with dread, consider the other benefits to giving up:

- As I mentioned earlier caffeine stimulates the release of cortisol from the adrenal gland. When there is too much cortisol in the body, it starts to have a negative effect on the levels of Estrogen and Progesterone circulating, causing an even bigger imbalance in hormone levels, leading to a worsening of menopausal symptoms.

- According to Patrick Holford (leading nutrition expert), Caffeine also increases levels of homocysteine in the body (a protein which is harmful when levels are high). High homocysteine levels increases your risk of getting many health disorders including heart disease, stroke, diabetes, Alzheimer's disease, some cancers and Osteoporosis; conditions already associated with Menopause.

- The side effects of caffeine such as insomnia, headaches and irritability are also symptoms of

Menopause, so it makes sense that if you drink caffeinated drinks, these symptoms will worsen.

- In a time when you may be struggling to maintain or lose weight, high fat, sugar-laced coffee drinks such as cappuccinos or lattes can account for many hidden calories. As well as this, for many people having a coffee / tea break can also mean having something sweet with it. When having healthier drinks such as herbal or fruit teas, you are less likely to associate having something sweet with it, thereby reducing the temptation and your calorie intake.

- Drinking too much tea, coffee or caffeinated energy drinks doesn't count towards hydration – they flush water out of your body causing dehydration, so drinking lots of these definitely just make things a whole lot worse.

- Bladder problems may have become an issue for you since reaching peri-menopause, as the reduction in Oestrogen can reduce the effectiveness of the muscles of the bladder and urinary tract, causing symptoms of:
  - o Urinary frequency - needing to go to the toilet regularly

       o   Urgency – when the urge to pee comes it is virtually impossible to suppress it, and you have to run to the toilet

Caffeine can also stimulate bladder activity, which worsens the symptoms of frequency and urgency you're already experiencing.

Alcohol & The Menopause

I don't want to be the complete party pooper and take all your fun away, but if the symptoms of Menopause are causing you great distress and suffering, and you're not enjoying life currently, then reducing your alcohol intake or cutting it out completely may turn out to be the best move you'll ever make towards feeling better physically, mentally and emotionally. If you are genuinely interested in managing your Menopause naturally, you'll find this is a small sacrifice for a great gain, and it may just be short-term until you get your symptoms under control.

My suggestion is to give alcohol a break for at least a 4-week trial period. I recommend keeping a diary during this period of time documenting your symptoms, especially the frequency and severity of hot flashes and of your general mood (including episodes of depression, anxiety, restlessness, nervousness and anger), as these are the two areas where you will notice the biggest improvement.

If after the 4 weeks you notice an improvement in your symptoms, then it's a no-brainer. If not, then I suggest you make your own decision whether you want to resume your old habit. To help you make an informed decision, I've outlined below some of the effects alcohol has on our bodies, our brain and our health.

As we grow older, our body finds it harder to process and metabolize alcohol, so we may have higher blood alcohol levels for longer periods of time than a younger person who has consumed the same amount and type of alcohol as you. Normally when we drink alcohol, it is diluted by the water in our bodies, but women have less water than men do, so it's less dilute. Therefore it will have a greater effect on the body, so women become more easily impaired, and it makes women more susceptible to alcohol related illnesses.

Alcohol destroys your ability to digest anything else. It irritates and alters your body, and radically destroys the amount of oxygen in your brain. You get "drunk" because of the low levels of oxygen reaching your brain. This happens because your body is actively

89

trying to restrict the flow of alcohol-soaked blood to the brain, in order to preserve it from this destructive poison.

Drinking alcohol weakens your immune system; it damages your brain and your central nervous system; your liver, your pancreas and your gallbladder; it increases your odds of diabetes and liver cancer, can lead to strokes, can cause ulcers in the esophagus and stomach, and wreaks havoc with your digestive system. Over the long term, drinking can actually shrink the frontal lobes of your brain and cause dementia. Alcohol makes it harder for your digestive tract to absorb nutrients and B vitamins or control bacteria.

If you do feel the need to have one, the current recommendation, is one drink per day. That equates to:
- 350mls of beer (12 ounces), OR
- 150mls of wine (5 ounces), OR
- 45mls distilled spirits, such as vodka, gin, rum, whisky, or brandy (1.5 ounces).

Flavonoids, (naturally occurring substances in food that come from plants) and other antioxidants found in red wine may help lower the formation of plaque on arteries. Rather than resorting to red wine though, you can get the same benefits from grapes or grape juice.

There is some research that suggests alcohol may help raise HDL cholesterol (good cholesterol) and reduce the risk of blood clots and heart disease, however the evidence is not strong enough to support these beliefs, so it's best to keep alcohol to a minimum.

Alcohol and weight management

The body is unable to store alcohol, so we automatically process it immediately. Therefore while the calories taken in by alcohol are being utilized or processed, the calories taken in by food become surplus to requirement and are therefore converted into fat, to be stored in the body (usually around the middle) until they are needed at a later time. This is the reason alcohol is not recommended if you are trying to lose a weight, at the very least alcohol slows down weight loss, and at most it contributes to weight gain.

Sugary mixed drinks or cocktails are especially bad if you are trying to manage weight issues. They spell double trouble; the alcohol sidetracks your fat burning mechanisms while the sugar spikes insulin (the hormone that tells your body to store fat). When weight watching, beer can become your enemy, as it contains gluten and refined carbohydrates. While there are gluten free beers, they're hard to find, and you're still feeding your body refined carbohydrates. Many studies reveal that gluten contributes to lots more ailments than celiac disease alone. A gluten-free diet has been shown to reduce inflammation, weight gain and insulin resistance, which is a major contributor in the onset of obesity and type-2 diabetes. If you feel the need to have that beer, choose the organic gluten-free variety.

Alcohol may also prevent the conversion of good fats (Omega 6) into substances that reduce inflammation within the body. So while you might be eating a healthy diet, you may not be getting the benefits from it if you're flushing out the good fats with alcohol. If you've taken healthy steps to optimize your nutrition by taking multi vitamin and multi mineral supplements, alcohol un-do's your good work as it depletes your storage of vitamin B and blocks the absorption of Vitamin C in the body, rendering your supplements pretty much useless!

Alcohol and hot flashes

Just as there are numerous theories on the causes of hot flashes, so too there are theories on why drinking alcohol increases the intensity and severity of hot flashes. We do know from research that as the liver tries to metabolize alcohol, it can only do this at a rate of 1 unit per hour. If you consume alcohol at a faster rate than this the excess alcohol in the blood stream can cause widening of blood vessels. When blood vessels near the skin widened, the skin becomes warm and this triggers the sweat glands to produce sweat, thereby facilitating hot flashes. Drinking a small amount of alcohol (at a rate of one unit per hour or less) may not induce a hot flash, but drinking larger amounts may lead to an accumulation of alcohol in the system that may continue to dilate blood vessels after drinking has stopped, causing night sweats. In women already prone to hot flashes, alcohol consumption could easily trigger one. If hot flashes are a particularly difficult symptom for you to get control over, then do the trial period I suggested earlier and see how you get on.

Alcohol and mental health

Alcohol is known to reduce serotonin (your happy hormone) levels in the brain, while raising cortisol levels. This in combination with fluctuations in hormone levels can trigger depression, anxiety, and panic attacks. All of which contribute to rising stress levels in your body, which in turn increases your risk of cardiovascular problems. If you've been unsuccessful in managing depressive symptoms using natural treatments and your depression needs to be treated with prescribed anti-depressants, alcohol also reduces their effectiveness. Prescribed anti-depressants and alcohol are a poor combination. When the liver is trying to metabolize the medication, it can't cope with the added pressure of alcohol on the system, causing you to get drunk faster, and enhancing the other negative effects of alcohol, giving you the hangover from hell.

Alcohol and Sleep

Alcohol produces both stimulant and sedating effects in humans, much to the surprise of many people, who often say they have a drink or two in the evening to help them relax and unwind. While alcohol may have this effect in the short term, its stimulant effect of raised heart rate lingers on long after you've gone to bed. This causes restlessness and interrupted sleep, as well as night sweats, leaving you feeling drained instead of refreshed the following morning. If you're experiencing symptoms of depression (low mood, and lacking in motivation), sleep deprivation can worsen the symptoms, since feeling tired all the time also reduces your drive and motivation.

Our memory and other aspects of brain functioning are all supported by a good night's sleep. During normal sleep our brains process all the activities of the day, and all information is recorded and backed up in our memory bank, similar to a computer (only much better!). With the symptoms of reduced Estrogen levels, hot flashes, nights sweats and sleep disturbances, this back up process is hugely hindered, leading to poor memory and an inability to concentrate. Therefore if you reduce your alcohol intake not only will your sleep improve, but you are also proactively managing the night sweats which in turn boosts your overall performance each day. This added up over time leads to a more energetic and fulfilling life.

Alcohol and Osteoporosis

More than two drinks per day interferes with calcium metabolism. Alcohol has a diuretic effect, that is, it causes the kidneys to flush out more water than usual from the body. This reduces the body's ability to absorb the minerals Calcium & Magnesium. These essential nutrients are necessary for bone health, so reducing their levels in your body leaves you more susceptible to breaking bones and Osteoporosis. The body needs

Vitamin D to help it make use of the calcium you take in through food. Alcohol has a negative impact on vitamin D metabolism, making it hard for your body to absorb calcium, increasing your risk of developing fragile bones and Osteoporosis.

Alcohol and Cancer

Reduce your alcohol intake to just one per day to significantly reduce your chances of developing certain cancers such as breast, esophageal, bowel, liver, mouth or larynx; all of which have been shown to occur less in women who don't drink at all. Why not weigh up the benefit versus the symptom control when it comes to deciding whether to cut alcohol out of your diet completely or not? If you are serious about maintaining good health, I feel the benefits of not drinking at all far outweigh the short-term pleasure of indulgence.

The rule of thumb = if you currently don't drink don't start, and if you do drink, maintain your intake at a low level.

By the way, a lot of beers are laden with high fructose corn syrup, artificial flavors and toxic ingredients such as airplane de-icing liquid, caramel coloring, propylene glycol, MSG (an *excitotoxin* that can cause brain damage, nervous disorders, and cause radical hormone fluctuations), GMO's, fish bladders, stabilizers like carrageenan that are linked to intestinal inflammation, and a host of other carcinogens. A lot of the American beer companies are not even using fermentation anymore, which essentially means you are not even drinking beer. Some beer manufactures are not even using real hops. They have a patent on something called *tetrahops*, which is a synthetic chemical that mimics hop flavor (which is significantly *cheaper* to produce). The caramel coloring often used is a carcinogen proven to cause liver tumors, lung tumors, and thyroid tumors in rats and mice. But it doesn't matter, since advertising will make consumers buy anything.

Shocking: *The manufacturers are not obliged to list all their ingredients on their packaging.* Stay away from alcohol – you don't really know *what* they put in those products.

Chapter 6

Key No. 4: Sleep & De-Stress

Your body needs rest. This is obvious of course, but you would be surprised at how many people in Western societies burn the candle at both ends. The motto *"Work Hard, Play Harder"*, or *"Work Hard, Party Harder"* is a recipe for burnout and crippling health problems by the time you reach your forties.

You're well aware at this stage that Menopause is not just about hormone levels dropping and their effect on the reproductive system, it causes a huge cascade of other changes throughout the body. For some, the most troublesome symptom of menopause is hot flashes, for others it is lack of sleep, and the knock on effects of sleep deprivation.

Women are more likely to experience sleep disturbances in the **Menopausal** period than at other times of life. Poor quality sleep is one of the most common complaints amongst Menopausal women, of whom 25–50% report sleep difficulties, compared to some 15% of the general population.

The exact reasons why sleep disturbances are more prevalent in Menopausal women are not well understood. It's still unclear how sleep disturbances are associated with the **hormonal** changes of Menopause. While hormonal changes are thought to play a role, they are most likely one of many factors contributing to the age-related increase in sleep disturbances that occur in both women and men.

To make some sense as to why sleep and stress may have become a problem for you now, let's talk about the science-y bit first...

During the time of transition through Menopause, the ovaries are producing less Estrogen and Progesterone and more Follicle stimulating hormone (FSH) and Lutenising Hormone (LH). During peri-menopause, lack of ovulation leads to significant drops in Progesterone.

Lowered levels of Progesterone and Estrogen, have a big impact on sleep. Progesterone has a sedative effect due to its stimulation of benzodiazepine receptors, which have anti-anxiety or sedative effects on the brain. You may recall (if you've had a pregnancy) the extreme fatigue you experienced in early pregnancy. This was due to the high Progesterone levels circulating throughout your body. During Peri-menopause the exact opposite is happening. Low levels of Progesterone, which is one of the most common hormone issues associated with peri-menopause, contribute hugely to sleep disturbances.

The effects of Estrogen are a little more complex; it has been shown that low Estrogen levels reduce our REM (rapid eye movement) part of the sleep cycle, which means our sleep quality is poorer. Lowered Estrogen levels also increase the frequency of waking from sleep, leaving you feeling as if you've not slept a wink all night, even when you have.

Estrogen also affects regulation of body temperature, and with reduced Estrogen levels you know you are prone to hot flashes; the discomfort of the hot flash or night sweat in combination with the effects mentioned above all lead to poor sleep quality and quantity.

During Peri-menopause and after Menopause, the adrenal glands and fat cells become the main source of

Estrogen production. A substance called Androstenedione, produced by the adrenal glands, is converted to Estrone in the fat cells. This is one of the reasons why women naturally increase body fat during this time and why leaner women may have more symptoms during the menopause transition.

In addition, several studies have shown that higher levels of Lutenising hormone (LH) also lead to sleep disturbances. Lutenising hormone is produced by the pituitary gland and is the hormone that also leads to ovulation during the child bearing years. In Menopause, when ovulation does not occur the body produces even more LH. It is thought that raised levels of LH concentrations happens immediately before waking episodes in menopausal women and that these surges are associated with increased body temperature and sleep disturbance.

Estrogen has a balancing effect on a number of neurotransmitters including 'the happy hormone' - Serotonin. Serotonin production declines with age, and at any age its abundance can be compromised further by stress. Low levels of Serotonin are most commonly manifested by depressed mood, anxiety and insomnia. Low Estrogen levels in the body also reduce production of the anti-anxiety neurotransmitter gamma-

Aminobutyric acid (commonly referred to as GABA), leading to increased anxiety.

As if all of this going on in the body outlined above wasn't enough to contend with, during Peri-menopause women also suffer with high levels of the stress hormone cortisol, which as mentioned previously is our fight or flight hormone! You can imagine with your body in fight or flight mode, it would be impossible to sleep, even when you're feeling exhausted. In the normal course of the day, our cortisol levels are high in the mornings when we need to get up and go, and usually fall towards evening, allowing the body to rest and sleep.

Our cortisol levels rise when we are stressed, and in today's world, with stressful situations abounding (deadlines, traffic, etc.) you can see how our cortisol levels can remain elevated for long periods of time into the evening, causing interruptions' in the natural sleep cycle, which leads on to chronic fatigue and insomnia. Raised cortisol levels also cause physical symptoms of rapid heart rate, palpitations (feeling like your heart will jump out of your chest), acute anxiety attacks and panic attacks.

Alongside the Estrogen receptors present in the breasts, womb and ovaries, as you would expect, there are also Estrogen receptors in women's bones, brain, blood vessels, central nervous system and skin. So it is not surprising that changes are experienced in all these areas when Estrogen levels decline. Hot flashes are the most debilitating symptom of the Menopause and they contribute to insomnia, irritability, poor concentration, loss of memory and even depression in some instances; causing varying degrees of stress for most women.

With Menopause, the body is ageing, and the prevalence of diseases that might potentially adversely impact sleep increase. These include:

- Depression
- Anxiety
- Arthritis
- Diabetes
- Fibromyalgia
- Sleep related breathing difficulties, such as sleep apnea.

Also, the incidence of snoring and awakening in partners' increases as you age and may create even further sleep disturbances.

Chronic insomnia can also contribute to physical

conditions such as heart disease, high blood pressure, and other lasting medical conditions. It also impacts job performance, your safety and your overall quality of life.

With all these changes occurring due to changes in your body and hormone levels, is it any wonder you're feeling *'tired and wired'*?

Don't Resort to Dangerous Prescription Sleeping Pills!

I know when you're feeling so fatigued and sleep deprived you'd do anything to get a good night's sleep. Please don't give in to the temptation when you are at such a low ebb to resort to sleeping pills. You can fool yourself by saying, "it's just for a short time to get me over the hump, once I've had a few good sleeps, I won't use them anymore". This is the start of the slippery slope to dependence on sleeping pills. You may say I'm exaggerating, but the stats speak for themselves:

- In 2012, 60 million Americans filled prescriptions for sleeping pills, up from 46 million in 2006 (as reported in The New York Times).
- In 2015 15.3 million public health prescriptions in the UK were made for sleep medication.

105

- Patients in England alone received 5.4m prescriptions for Zopiclone and 2.8m for Temazepam, the two most popular sleeping pills.
- The Economic and Social Research Institute UK, published numbers relating to prescribed sleeping pills, stating that; 1 in 10 people in Britain suffer from insomnia, yet the only treatment offered in most doctors' surgeries is a course of sleeping tablets. Known to increase as people grow older, insomnia is often connected with a long-term illness. However, among these patients, doctors have found sleeping drugs bring only minor benefits, and pose a significant risk of harm.

According to a study published in the British Medical Journal (BMJ), receiving prescriptions for hypnotics (sleeping pills) was associated with a greater than threefold increased hazard of death, even when prescribed less than 18 pills per year. This association held in separate analyses for several commonly used sleeping pills and for newer shorter-acting drugs. Control of selective prescription sleeping pills for people in poor health did not explain the observed excess mortality.

If you've previously considered yourself a cool, calm and collected individual, you can see how with the effect of all the hormone changes going on in your body, why you may not be enjoying being the person you once were, and it's NOT 'all in your head'. The good news is YOU can manage this effectively, and WITHOUT prescription medication.

Managing Sleep

When your sleep is disturbed you naturally feel tired and drained the next day. This reduces your ability to cope, which increases your stress levels, which disturbs your sleep and the vicious cycle continues! So how do you break the cycle?

Firstly, take on the tips I gave earlier in Key No. 1 on food to help balance the blood sugars. Often hot flashes are confused with adrenaline surges, caused by low blood sugars.

1. Avoid foods with a high-glycemic index, which will cause your blood sugar to spike (processed foods, sugar, any meals or snacks containing refined carbohydrates - white rice, white pasta and white flour - soft drinks, fruit juices,

chocolate, biscuits, etc.) Chose whole, unprocessed, foods without added sugar.

2. Eat regular meals, especially breakfast. When you eat a good breakfast, it sets your blood sugars on the right track for the day, so eat a good one.

3. Have some protein, fat and fiber with each meal. These three components will keep your blood sugars on an even keel.

4. A SMALL (don't be tempted to go for second helpings!!) savory snack before bedtime will help to maintain normal blood sugars and prevent an adrenaline surge during the night.

5. Consider taking a chromium supplement. 200 micrograms daily helps your body use insulin better and reduces sugar cravings.

When it comes to dietary fiber, we often think of insoluble fiber such as bran, and although it will improve regularity and contribute to good bowel health, it won't stabilize your blood sugar. Soluble fiber is much more effective at balancing blood sugars, and is found in whole, unprocessed fruit, veggies, legumes, nuts and seeds. Soluble fiber absorbs water to form a natural fiber gel in the stomach. The gel combines with sugar to release it more slowly into the blood stream, reducing the impact on blood sugar levels.

108

Food can be disruptive right before sleep. Stay away from large meals close to bedtime, as this stimulates the digestive system and can keep you awake. Not to mention it may trigger symptoms of heartburn or other digestive symptoms. Also remember that chocolate has caffeine in it, which is a brain stimulant.

As discussed in chapter 3, moderate exercise (does not have to be strenuous) for 30 minutes per day on average, is a great way to reduce stress as it helps your body burn off the stress hormones adrenaline and cortisol. This leaves you feeling more relaxed at bedtime and less likely to wake during the night. Exercise also stimulates Endorphin release into the blood stream, which reduces the symptoms of depression, which is known to cause sleep disturbances.

Vigorous exercise is best carried out in the morning or late afternoon. Whereas a relaxing exercise such as Yoga or Pilates done before bed is great to initiate a restful night's sleep.

Sleep Hygiene

'Sleep hygiene' is the term used to describe good sleep habits. Considerable research has gone into developing guidelines and tips designed to enhance good sleep. While implementing the suggestions mentioned in earlier chapters, have a look at the sleep hygiene tips below, which may provide long-term solutions to sleep difficulties.

Quit - or at a minimum - reduce Stimulants (see Key No. 3: Good Hydration)

Avoid stimulants such as caffeine, nicotine and alcohol completely if possible, or too close to bedtime. While alcohol is well known to speed the onset of sleep, it disrupts sleep in the second half of the night as the body begins to break down the alcohol, and stimulates the body to wake early.

Get good exposure to natural light

This is particularly important for you as you get older since you may become slower, and venture outside less frequently than children and young adults. Light exposure helps maintain a healthy sleep-wake cycle.

Light tells the brain it is time to wake up. The light helps to regulate your biological clock and keep it on track. This internal clock is located in the brain and keeps time (similarly to the clock we use ourselves). By staying up later and, more importantly, getting up later, we put our internal clock out of sync, which means we may have trouble getting to sleep and waking up when we need to.

To keep the body in sync, we need to reset our clock each day so that it stays compatible with the external time of night and day. Exposing ourselves to light, especially in the mornings, appears to accomplish this resetting. Research has shown that people who are deprived of light for long periods of time (and so do not have their biological clocks reset) experience dramatic disruptions in their sleep, temperature and hormone cycles.

Many factors affect our biological clock, but light appears to be the most important. The timing of this sunlight exposure is also crucial; the body clock is most responsive to sunlight in the early morning, between 6 a.m. and 8:30 a.m. Exposure to sunlight later does not provide the same benefit. The type of light also matters, as does the length of exposure. Direct sunlight outdoors for at least half an hour produces the most benefit. Our indoor lighting in a normal home or office has little effect.

Quit or reduce your smoking habit

As if there weren't enough good reasons to quit smoking, here's another one!!

In 2008, a clinical study looking at the effects of cigarette smoking on sleep was carried out at The Johns Hopkins University, in Baltimore, Maryland, and was later published in 'Chest', the journal of the American College of Chest Physicians. The study showed a number of interesting findings; an analysis of brain-wave activity showed that compared with nonsmokers, smokers on average had a higher percentage of light sleep and a lower percentage of deep sleep.

The researchers also found that the findings on brain wave activity were reflected in how smokers felt after their night's sleep. Lack of restful sleep was reported by 22.5% of the smokers, compared with only 5.0% of the nonsmokers. Smokers also had more complaints of feeling unrested after the night of sleep.

The direct effects of smoking on sleep seen in this study demonstrate smokers are not getting a restful sleep. This has ramifications for them on a daily basis; they're going to be tired the next day and most likely they will have diminished level of alertness, having direct effects on their daily living.

The study authors reported that as the nicotine levels in the body continue to drop after 2 hours, people experienced impaired sleep quality, due to nicotine withdrawal. If you find that your menopausal symptoms include sleep disturbances, try quitting the fags. You'll notice a substantial improvement in the quality of your sleep within weeks.

Cognitive Behavioural therapy or CBT

CBT for Insomnia, often called CBT-I, is an approved method for treating sleep disturbances or insomnia without resorting to sleeping pills. CBT is aimed at changing sleep habits and scheduling factors, as well as working with a person's attitudes and beliefs towards sleep and insomnia, which often serve to galvanize sleep difficulties.

Behavioural therapies are the foundation of long-term improvements to sleep quality. They may be used alone or in addition to other treatments. Sleep-enhancing behavioural therapies such as sleep hygiene as outlined here, or other techniques used in CBT all play a role in relieving sleep disturbances. Women with comorbid psychological symptoms such as stress and anxiety would certainly benefit from CBT.

Set up a regular relaxing bedtime routine

You can't control when the sun shines, but you can control the level of stress in your life. Try to avoid emotionally upsetting conversations and activities before retiring to bed. For instance, if you find a particular friend is a negative person and can be an energy drain on you, avoid speaking to that person (if possible) before retiring to bed. Instead speak to them in the morning or afternoon, to minimize their effect on your mood and sleep. Try not to dwell on, or bring your problems to bed. Some people find writing out a 'to do' list, and getting it out of their head and onto paper, also reduces the clutter in their head, allowing them to relax.

Associate your bedroom with sleep

- It's not a good idea to use your bed to watch TV, listen to the radio or read.
- Maintain regular times both for getting to bed and getting up from bed, including weekends.
- Establish a regular, relaxing bedtime routine such as taking a bath or listening to relaxing music (BEFORE heading to the bedroom).
- Create restful surroundings that may induce sleep such as; a dark, quiet and comfortable

room, with a comfortable temperature – not too hot or too cold.

- Ensure you have a comfortable bed, mattress and pillows.
- Sleep with a window open to allow fresh air in and use light covers. Remaining cool during the night can lead to better quality and more restful sleep.
- Apart from sleep, the only other activity in the bedroom recommended is sex.
- Use a relaxing activity such as; massage, meditation, breathing exercises or listening to relaxation techniques/music for 20 to 30 minutes, particularly right before bedtime may help you fall into a deeper sleep faster - and that usually means better quality rest.

Natural remedies to promote sleep

- Herbal teas of **valerian root**, passionflower or chamomile taken 45 minutes before **bedtime** might induce a deeper and more restful sleep.
- **Isoflavones** (plant compounds that contain a weak form of Estrogen called Phytoestrogen) found in Soya based products, chickpeas and lentils, were reported in one study to improve

sleep quality and reduce the frequency of insomnia.

- Red clover (contains Isoflavones) has also demonstrated in clinical studies to improve sleep in post-menopausal women. One study reported a combination of Isoflavones, lactobacilli, Magnolia bark extract, **magnesium**, vitamin D3 and **calcium** decreased the severity and frequency of sleep disturbances, as well as hot flashes.

- Vitamin B complex and Magnesium work directly on the adrenal glands and help calm the body down. B vitamins are often known as "stress" vitamins because of their beneficial effect, and Magnesium is known as "nature's tranquillizer".

Once a good night's sleep has been obtained, the benefits of this go far beyond just feeling refreshed the following day. It has hugely positive effects on other common **symptoms of menopause such as energy levels, depression mood swings.**

- Sleep helps our bodies to regulate our emotions, so we are better able to deal with small emotional upsets (possibly caused by fluctuating hormone levels) without overreacting by snapping at someone, or bursting into tears.

- Better weight management. This happens on 2 levels; firstly on a physical level, if you are feeling tired you're less likely to have the energy and drive to get out and exercise, (even though it's one thing that would help you sleep better). Secondly when you sleep, you produce more of the hormone Leptin, which helps you to feel full. When you're sleep deprived, your Leptin levels drop, causing you to feel hungry and crave high fat and high calorie foods.

- Clearer thinking – while you sleep your brain is working in other ways, 'backing up' all you learnt and memorized in the preceding days. Your brain then works more efficiently when you wake, as the 'backup' process has been completed.

- Stronger immunity - research conducted shows that people who got on average 8 hours sleep per night were much less likely to pick up the common cold than those who got an average of 7 hours or less.

- Less pain - many studies have shown a link between sleep loss and lower pain threshold. Of course being in pain can make it hard to sleep. Research has been conducted demonstrating good sleep patterns can supplement medication for pain.

Learn How to De-stress

As we mentioned earlier, in order to improve our sleep we need to break the vicious cycle of being 'tired but wired'. We do this by adapting some of the strategies I've suggested above, and managing our stress levels proactively. Learning how to de-stress will be the best present you can ever give your self – be generous to YOU.

Stress has your body in 'fight or flight' mode, ready to run away or fight off danger. During 'fight or flight' mode, blood flow is focused on your arms and legs, and adrenaline and cortisol flood your body. This shuts down your digestion; toxicity accumulates, and impacts your general health.

Stress can physically damage your heart muscle. Stress damages your heart because stress hormones (Adrenaline and Cortisol) increase your heart rate and constrict your blood vessels. At the same time it prepares to thicken the blood, in case it needs to prevent hemorrhage in the event of an injury. This forces your heart to work harder and increases your blood pressure. Stress weakens your immune system, and chronic stress is a major contributor to premature aging (wrinkles, weak muscles, poor eyesight and more).

Stress has also been linked to cancer, lung disease, fatal accidents, suicide and cirrhosis of the liver.

How to reduce your stress levels:

- Make a list of the things that stress you out at the moment and examine each one in depth to come up with ways to deal with it.
- Find your purpose and do what you truly love. What is your passion? What is your unique ability?
- Simplify your life; eliminate the clutter in your life.
- Meditate for 15-20 minutes twice a day.
- Adopt a spiritual understanding of life. Let go of the illusion that anything in the Universe is not exactly as it should be…
- Educate yourself about wealth creation and master your finances – keep a budget, spend less than you earn and invest the difference.

- Turn down the noise; minimize your time spent watching TV and using the Internet to help reduce aural and mental clutter in your life.
- Plan ahead and make sure you're always on time or at least 15 minutes early for appointments. This helps reduce stress that can arise from traffic or underestimating travel times. Ultimately, it allows you to slow down and focus before an event.

Eat in a relaxed state.

Turn the TV off and eat slowly, chewing your food well. Focus only on your food, this means getting rid of all other distractions. When you eat, make sure you do JUST that. DO NOT eat on the run. Sit down and eat your food to help you notice how much of what you're actually eating. Have your smallest meal in the late afternoon or early evening, NOT the other way around.

Meditate

Close to 600 scientific studies have shown that meditation brings distinct improvements in health, including a marked reduction in stress and anxiety levels, improved sleep, increased vitality and energy levels; the ageing process slows down, blood pressure normalizes, chronic illnesses decrease and creativity and the ability to focus and think clearly increases.

REVERSAL OF AGING PROCESS
through the Transcendental Meditation program

PHYSIOLOGY	Through aging	Through TM	PSYCHOLOGICAL	Through aging	Through TM
Blood pressure	↑	↓	Susceptibility to stress	↑	↓
Auditory threshold	↑	↓	Behavioral rigidity	↑	↓
Near-point vision	↑	↓	Learning ability	↓	↑
Cardiovascular efficiency	↓	↑	Memory	↓	↑
Cerebral blood flow	↓	↑	Creativity	↓	↑
Homeostatic recovery	↓	↑	Intelligence	↓	↑
			HEALTH		
BIOCHEMISTRY			Cardiovascular disease	↑	↓
Cholesterol concentration	↑	↓	Hypertension	↑	↓
Hemoglobin cencentration	↓	↑	Asthma (severity)	↑	↓
			Insomnia	↑	↓
MIND-BODY COORDINATION			Depression	↑	↓
Reaction time	↑	↓	Immune system efficiency	↓	↑
Sensory-motor performance	↓	↑	Quality of sleep	↓	↑

Chapter 7

Key No. 5: Manage Your Mind

The physiological effects of Menopause are widely known and talked about; hot flashes, night sweats, painful heavy periods, digestive issues and sleep disturbances to mention just a few! For reasons unknown, possibly due to the stigma or the possibility that other people might think you're going mad, the effects of Menopause on the brain (both psychological and emotional) are less talked about. However they are very real issues for many women, even more so than the physiological ones.

If you consider yourself a generally good humored, well-balanced and optimistic person, but recently you've noticed you're ready to take the head off someone for the slightest thing, or you're feeling down with no obvious reason for feeling this way, and your likely to break down in tears at any moment, then you're most likely experiencing the effects of lowered hormone levels on the brain.

Many women I have spoken with, when probed about how it's affecting their mood, talk about the completely irrational mood swings they experience, feeling down or blue with no apparent reason and or scary anxiety levels, on a scale never experienced before.

Be reassured you are not "losing it" or imagining it. Unfortunately it's very real, and yet again the hormones are to blame. These are all symptoms of fluctuating hormone levels. As you progress through the menopause, your body doesn't just reduce the production of hormones Estrogen, Progesterone and Testosterone, instead your body erratically produces them, causing low levels one minute and soaring levels the next! Is it any wonder you don't know where your brain is half the time, never mind what it's doing or thinking?

It's most likely that Progesterone levels are the first to fall. This can lead to symptoms of irritability including anxiety, brain fog and mood swings. Brain fog includes symptoms of confusion, memory loss and lack of focus, or fuzzy thinking. You would be forgiven for thinking you're developing Alzheimer's, but forgetfulness caused by Menopause is not believed to make you more likely to develop Alzheimer's. Once Menopause is over, brain function usually returns to normal. Since the functions of Progesterone include reducing anxiety and increasing sleepiness, in its absence it's no surprise that we suffer sleep disturbances as discussed in the last chapter, as well as anxiety, both affecting mental wellbeing.

Following on from lowered Progesterone levels, we may experience a fall in Testosterone levels. This can cause diminished sex drive and low mood or depression. Then comes the drop in Estrogen, which further compounds the mood swings, depression and brain fog, as well as possibly causing headaches and decreased energy. Estrogen is believed to help raise levels of acetylcholine, which has a positive influence on our memory, and conversely lowered Estrogen levels lead to lowered levels of acetylcholine, hence the memory difficulties.

Estrogen blocks the breakdown of Serotonin and noradrenalin. The knock on effect of lowered Estrogen levels is lowered Serotonin (The Happy Hormone) and Noradrenalin (not really hormones more neuro-transmitters). This goes towards explaining why women are more prone to depression during Peri-menopause and thereafter.

What we consider to be symptoms of Menopause can also be symptoms of low Serotonin levels, such as:
- Emotional outbursts - tearfulness, or feelings of despair
- Feeling tense, irritable, angry or resentful
- Tendency towards comfort eating
- Brain fog - poor memory or concentration
- Low energy levels
- Sleep disturbances
- Low libido
- Depression
- Anxiety

Serotonin is a key influencer in our mood. Research has shown that there are numerous reasons for low Serotonin levels, one of which is low Estrogen levels.

There are other causes of low serotonin levels such as:
1. Too much stress
2. Not enough light
3. Not enough exercise
4. Not enough vitamins and minerals especially Vitamin C and folic acid.

5. Lack of the amino acid Tryptophan, which helps manufacture Serotonin.

There are 2 other dimensions possibly affecting your emotional health and well-being at this time:

1. Most women are experiencing other Menopausal symptoms in tandem with the emotional symptoms. These include hot flashes, night sweats, fatigue, sleep disturbances, urogenital problems such as difficulty getting to the toilet on time and pain during sex, all symptoms which can cause additional stress and anxiety.

2. Symptoms occur in midlife - when other things in your life may be going on for you, affecting your mood, such as:

- Empty nest syndrome
- Fear of, or reluctance to age
- Other health problems
- Early retirement
- Relationship issues (which can occur at any time)
- Death of loved ones (close friends, partner or parent)

Any of which further compounds the effects the fluctuating hormone levels have on your emotional state, hence the term - 'Mid-Life Crisis'!

The risk of depression appears to be higher during Peri-menopause - when hormone levels are changing - than during Post-menopause, when Estrogen and Progesterone levels are low but stable.

The change in hormone levels (either a rise or a fall) means your brain must deal with it. When the change is small, the brain can sort it out with relative ease, and you hardly notice any symptoms. When the change is more dramatic, the sudden change disrupts an entire chain of events, causing a lot of the symptoms mentioned above.

The Study of Women Across a Nation (better known as the SWAN study, conducted in the USA and published in 2011), showed that cognitive decline is common, and that it can be more difficult to learn new things as you go through Menopause. The good news in this study is that Menopausal cognitive decline might be time-limited, so as you near the later stages of Menopause, you do get more clarity. The lead of the SWAN study, researcher Miriam Weber, Ph.D. said between one-third and two-thirds of women report forgetfulness and other memory difficulties during Peri-menopause and Menopause. However, just because we have the research to show that we are not alone, and we are not 'going mad', does not make it any less frustrating when trying to manage it.

A study published in Psychological Science in 2008 found that certain inherited genes seem to account for 50 percent of our happiness. But even if your natural tendency is to be more down than up, you can make choices that will help you experience a brighter, happier life.

Hormones and neurotransmitters moderate our feelings of wellbeing, and lifestyle factors affect them. Read on below to see how you can help yourself to boost the happy hormones and neurotransmitters.

Non-Hormonal Brain Protection

While the experts may produce conflicting reports on the mechanism of how Menopause affects the brain, they agree that taking care of the brain is the best defense against cognitive decline. Focus on taking the following steps to increase Serotonin levels. This then helps control some of the Menopausal symptoms you are experiencing, giving you back control of your emotions and leaving you feeling happier and much less stressed.

129

Step 1 – Use Key no. 1: Food

Blood sugar surges and drops add fuel to the fire when managing mood swings, irritability and depression. Implement the guidelines given in Key No. 1: Food to help balance your blood sugars, and balance your mood.

Step 2 – Use Key No. 2: Movement is Medicine

Do some physical activity for at least 30 minutes on most days of the week, preferably outdoors. Physical exercise stimulates the pituitary gland to produce Endorphins, while the thyroid gland stimulates production of Serotonin; production of these two chemicals is often correlated so that elevating Endorphin levels can produce a natural rise in Serotonin levels.

Step 3 - Recognize what's happening

Perhaps discuss the erratic feelings you're having with your partner (or close friend) so that they can better understand what you're going through. This may also help reduce your stress levels, which is the fourth step. Some women find it beneficial to keep a diary – this can help you identify what is a Menopausal symptom and what is more likely to be symptoms of anxiety and/or depression. If you find after keeping the diary for some days or weeks, and have implemented the steps outlined here, that you're still experiencing symptoms of anxiety and/or depression, perhaps a visit to your medical doctor would be advisable.

Step 4 – Use Key No. 4: De-stress
Stress reduction is important for everyone, but is particularly important for women in Menopause. As discussed in Key no. 4, when you experience stress your Cortisol levels increase and Serotonin levels drop, which in turn affect your hormone activity to such an extent that it can induce symptoms. Therefore reducing your levels of stress can also have the opposite beneficial effect.

It has been reported that women who took part in relaxation techniques saw a 30% reduction in their hot flashes, and a big drop in tension, anxiety and depression. They also reported less mood swings and felt their mood was much better overall. By doing something every day to reduce your stress, such as going for a short walk, doing some breathing exercises, or putting time aside to relax and unwind, it helps balance hormones, creating a positive effect on mood swings. It can also have the added benefit of giving you energy to deal with other challenges in your life.

I know your possibly saying, *'How can I relax when I'm feeling like this?'* It can be incredibly difficult to de-stress initially when your feelings of irritability, anxiety and low energy are at their worst. But by persisting with this every day, you will slowly learn to relax into it, and start to reap the benefits. If you have never been good at relaxing or taking time out it can be a real challenge to begin with, but once you keep doing something to help you relax, you will develop the habit, and it will then become easier over time – persistence pays.

The positive is: Reducing even small stresses in your life - or simply setting aside some time every day to relax and unwind - can not only affect hormone balance but have a dramatic effect on your mood swings.

Step 5 – Manage the outbursts
Now that you know you're not 'going mad" and you know the cause of the unusual feelings your experiencing, rather than attack straight away, try to step back and analyze what's happening and if feasible, let the moment pass. Chances are that your mood swing will also pass, and you'll have avoided the outburst. Sometimes if you don't spend energy fighting the feeling, you can feel better faster and calm down faster. Of course there are times when this is not

feasible or you need to deal with it immediately, in which case go right ahead!

Step 6 - Practice mindfulness

Before you say, *'Oh for God sake, she clearly hasn't a clue how bad I'm feeling at the moment, how on Earth does she expect me to practice mindfulness'*....Trust me, take a deep breath and read on. I was once that person who said I haven't a hope of being mindful, I don't know how to do it, I've never done it before and I'll probably never be able to master it. To my surprise, I have managed to learn the how, the why and the when. I won't claim to be a master at it yet, but I'm certainly taking baby steps towards it.

You see, although Mindfulness has been practiced for generations, it is a relatively new buzz word. It conjures up all sorts of fears and anxieties in people's imagination thinking *'I don't even know what it is never mind how to do it.'*

Mindfulness at its most basic level is just sitting, standing, or lying there and becoming aware of what's happening right NOW. The idea is to focus on what's going on inside – your breathing, your muscle tension, your heart rate, your eye movements... The whole idea of Mindfulness or 'being mindful' is to calm the brain

133

and quiet the mind so that you can fully relax. At the other end of the Mindfulness spectrum is meditation. Once you've mastered how to be mindful, you may progress to meditate, and reap the many benefits associated with it.

I highly recommend if you're suffering the symptoms of mood swings, stress, anxiety or depression that you learn Mindfulness. You will be amazed at how beneficial you find it. One of my coaching clients, a woman in her late 40's, was suffering really badly with hot flashes and anxiety relating to Menopause. Through my Menopause management program, she started to practice Mindfulness, and within 6 weeks of her starting she noticed a dramatic improvement in both her symptoms of hot flashes and anxiety.

Clinical studies examining the benefits of Mindfulness have discovered that women suffering with insomnia and hot flashes found that both these symptoms improved when compared with women with these symptoms who did not practice mindfulness.

A study from the University of California, Santa Barbara, found that meditation (AKA Mindfulness training), improves working memory and diminishes mind wandering—the two biggest brain problems women experience during Peri-menopause and Menopause. In the study, women completed a two-week Mindfulness course that involved daily meditation exercises.

According to another study published in the Journal of Mid-Life Health (2010), on the benefits of meditation and Yoga, meditation has been found to be associated with increased plasma melatonin levels and improved sleep quality, particularly if done in the evening before rest.

Step 7 – Consider Yoga or Pilates
Yoga
Again you may be saying, *'You've got to be kidding. I can hardly move, never mind practice yoga!'* Trust me; don't knock it until you've tried it.

The best part I found with Yoga is that you only do what you think or feel you're able to do. The Yoga teacher / instructor won't be expecting you to do hand stands or sit bow legged when you join a class. As my own Yoga teacher said, 'People who practice Yoga for years may never be able to touch their toes, and that's fine too.' You only do what you are able to do, so take that pressure off yourself immediately.

135

According to the study mentioned above *'Yoga and menopausal transition' published in the Journal of Mid-Life Health (2010),* Yoga has been utilized as a therapeutic tool to achieve positive health and control and cure many diseases. The exact mechanism as to how Yoga helps in various disease states is not known. There could be neuro-hormonal pathways with a selective effect in each pathological situation.

There have been multiple studies that have combined the many aspects of Yoga into a general Yoga session in order to investigate its effects on menopausal symptoms.

Some menopausal women find it difficult to overcome the symptom of reduced self-esteem and self-image. *Yoga* can be used as a form of exercise to overcome this issue. Yoga practice may provide a source of distraction from daily life and enhancement of self-esteem, helping women to focus on the simplicity of movement and forget about work responsibility and demands, and thus reduce anxiety and depression.

In this same study they found the integrated approach (that means movement along with breathing exercises and meditation) of Yoga therapy can improve hot flashes and night sweats. It can also improve cognitive functions such as remote memory, mental balance, attention and concentration.

A pilot study of Hatha Yoga treatment for Menopausal symptoms also showed improvement in Menopausal symptoms. Even eight weeks of an integrated approach to Yoga therapy resulted in better outcomes as compared to physical activity in reducing climacteric symptoms, perceived stress and neuroticism in Peri-menopausal women.

Pilates

Pilates can be of particular benefit during Peri-menopause, as it has so many facets to it that can alleviate symptoms. The gentle stretching and toning helps to relieve stress and reduce anxiety. A more rigorous Pilates workout can get the heart pumping faster for a sustained period (at least 20 minutes) which releases endorphins—the feel good hormone—into the bloodstream, reducing low mood or depressive symptoms. Also, as we need to concentrate on each move we make, this 'Mindfulness' helps to reduce stress and anxiety, helping us to feel more relaxed leading to a better night's sleep.

Step 8 – Develop a Positive Mental Attitude (PMA)

Your thoughts and feelings have a dramatic impact on

your health, so why not make it a positive effect?

Through my work as a health coach I like to empower my clients to make positive changes in their life. When women make decisions about managing their own health, and implement the options they've chosen that increases their self-esteem and their self-confidence, this empowers them to do even more for themselves.

In a clinical study on depression in Menopause, negative anticipation of Menopause seems to be associated with elevated rates of depression and physical symptoms of Menopause. Educational groups that help women learn what to expect during Menopause decreased anxiety, depression and irritability, both immediately after the group therapy and 1 year later. Based on this finding, *'fore-warned is fore-armed'*; if you research menopause and what to expect, you may minimize the negative aspects to it.

In 1998, a study showed that self-management programs using techniques designed to eliminate negative thought loops and promote positive emotional states can successfully decrease cortisol levels (McCraty and colleagues).

The truth is positive thinking doesn't mean ignoring the symptoms of Menopause; it instead helps you see them in a new light. Think about it; regardless of how you react to an external situation, the situation will still be the same. If being upset doesn't change the outcome of a past situation, wouldn't it serve you, and your health, to see the positives?

A positive mental attitude creates a mindset of enthusiasm and solutions. Instead of thinking about what can't be done, positive thinking allows you freedom to think of new ways to solve problems because you are not limited by fear of failure. When we are in a state of enthusiasm, we provide an open mind; we are in a state of allowance, openly accepting life and opportunity to flow to us.

What are the positive to be gained from menopause? Freedom from monthly periods, PMS and the fear of pregnancy can be remarkably liberating! It's important to take advantage of this wakeup call to say, *'let's make the most of this life'*. There is no *one* way, just *your* way, that's right for you.

Step 9 - Connect

According to Dr. Henry S. Lodge, MD, hundreds of studies confirm that isolation hurts us and connection heals us through the same basic, physical mechanisms as exercise and diet. Older people who have at least one close friend have cardiovascular systems that are younger by a series of objective measures than those of isolated people.

I'm sure you don't need to read the research papers to know that when we socialize with friends or family we feel better. So connect with the people around you; with family, friends, colleagues and neighbors; at home, work or in your local community. Think of these as the cornerstones of your life and invest time in developing them. Building these connections will support and enrich you every day.

It comes back to reducing the dreaded stress hormone cortisol. Meeting with friends or family can do more than distract you from your problems; their very presence may help temper your hormonal stress response. Simply anticipating laughter is enough to reduce cortisol levels by nearly half, according to researchers at Loma Linda University.

Feelings of isolation may prevent you from sharing what you're experiencing with friends or family members. You may find it easier to speak with a trained therapist who can help you cope with the challenges you're experiencing.

Chapter 8

Key No. 6: Support Supplements & Remedies

The great part of managing Menopause naturally is that you can take charge of it all yourself without reliance on doctors, drugs or other external influences. Use the keys to unlock your body from the intolerable symptoms you may be suffering.

Freedom from menopause naturally includes:
- Making lifestyle changes
- Adopting a healthy, hormone balancing diet
- Getting or maintaining physical fitness
- Maintaining adequate hydration
- Managing sleep and de-stressing
- Managing the mind
- Taking appropriate vitamins and mineral supplements
- Taking natural remedies to manage specific Menopausal symptoms

Supplements, Vitamins & Minerals

As we know, the 1st key to unlocking yourself from Menopausal mayhem is to eat a wide variety of healthy foods. Due to modern farming techniques, food processing methods and the effects of cooking, our food is often stripped of vitamins by the time it reaches our plates. Furthermore, the human body requires small amounts of about 25-30 minerals (14-16 of which are considered to be "essential") to maintain normal body function and good health. But due to modern dietary habits, and soils eroded by intensive agricultural practices, most of us are mineral deficient.

As we age our bodies become less efficient at absorbing nutrients from the food we eat; just at the very time we need the nutrients even more to help us maintain good health, hence the need for supplements.

Most vitamins require the presence of other nutrients to be utilized properly by the body. For this reason, it may be best to obtain vitamins from a whole food supplement or a multiple vitamin-mineral formula, rather than taking supplement forms of individual nutrients. The benefits we derive from taking these at this stage of life are endless; here are some to consider:

Managing Menopause

Multivitamin and mineral supplements are particularly beneficial during Peri-menopause to give us good baseline health, and to assist us in dealing with the symptoms we may be experiencing. For example, it's essential to take vitamin D when taking Calcium supplementation, as vitamin D is required for Calcium absorption from our digestive system. Magnesium is equally important as it renders vitamin D active to create the right environment to absorb Calcium from the gut. Vitamin B6 is essential to the syntheses of hemoglobin, which helps to prevent anemia, especially for those suffering heavy blood loss during menstruation.

Re-balance

Our nutrition boosts immunity and energy levels, especially if:

- o We take prescribed medications
- o We have recently fought off viral or bacterial infections
- o We have recently undergone surgery

Stress Management

The B vitamins, which include thiamine, niacin, B12 and folic acid are also known as the 'stress vitamins'). Some of the most common symptoms of vitamin B complex deficiency could be confused with symptoms

143

of Menopause. These include tension, anxiety, irritability, difficulty managing stress and poor concentration.

Fight disease
Multivitamin and mineral supplements support the body in the fight against diseases we become more susceptible to as we age, such as heart disease, diabetes, inflammatory conditions like arthritis, or fibromyalgia; as well as degenerative diseases such as Dementia, Alzheimer's Disease and Osteoporosis.

Brain food
Many clinical trials have demonstrated that taking a multi-vitamin & mineral supplement on a daily basis can result in improvements in memory. This is especially beneficial during Menopause when dropping hormone levels can cause us to suffer 'brain-fog'.

Mood Enhancers
Taking daily multivitamins and minerals have been shown through research to boost mood and emotional wellbeing. When our mood is better we manage our stress levels much better too, reducing nervous tension and anxiety.

Weight Management

Clinical research has also demonstrated that people with excess weight issues taking a daily multivitamin and mineral supplement were more successful in losing weight than those who did not. This makes perfect sense, because if your body is not getting all its essential vitamins and minerals, how can it work effectively to maintain the body in peak condition, including weight control. According to Patrick Holford, leading nutrition expert, our bodies require Zinc and Vitamin B6 to make Insulin, and Insulin's ability to control blood sugar levels is helped by Chromium, an essential mineral that, in helping to stabilize blood sugar levels, helps control weight. The body also needs the B vitamins, vitamin C and Magnesium to assist the body to convert Glucose into energy instead of into fat.

Improve Physical and Mental Condition

People who are stressed are less likely to keep track of their health and nutritional requirements. Daily multivitamin supplements can help you stay healthy, especially when you're under stress - when the body's ability to absorb vitamins and minerals is severely compromised. A daily intake of a good multivitamin supplement improves physical and mental health, boosts general bodily functions and promotes overall wellbeing. B3, B6, B12, Folic acid and Omega 3 & 6 are the keys to unlocking good brain health. The B vitamins and Folic acid are required to keep the brain from seizing up on you and they keep the essential neurotransmitters (dopamine, adrenaline, nor adrenaline and serotonin) fit and moving, to work effectively for you.

Prevents deficiency

The human body needs 13 essential vitamins. It is necessary to have the vitamins A, C, D, E, K, B complex (7) and B12 for the body to function properly. A deficiency of any of these vitamins can result in many issues, at its least – functioning below par; feeling tired and drained of energy at worst, which may result in illness and health complications. Therefore a daily intake of multivitamin and mineral supplements can prevent deficiencies arising, and lower the risk of illnesses.

Recommended support supplements & Remedies

Vitamin D3 (should be contained within your multivitamin)

Vitamin D3 is unique because it acquires hormone-like actions when it's converted to Calcitriol by the liver and kidneys. As a hormone, Calcitriol controls Phosphorus and Calcium metabolism, therefore promoting bone health, and reducing the risk of Osteoporosis. Vitamin D3 deficiency is linked to a surprising number of other health conditions such as depression, back pain, cancer, impaired immunity and macular degeneration (a condition of the eyes, leading to diminished vision and blindness).

Essential Oils & Fats - Omega 3 Supplements

Our body *needs* certain fats and oils. The 'Essential Oils', known as Omegas 3 and 6, are absolutely essential for every aspect of our health, from energy and stamina, to weight loss, brain function, heart health, the immune system, the skin, detoxification, digestion, and Menopause. Fats are an essential part of each and every cell and without them we would not be able to survive. Essential Fatty Acids that you absorb, for example from fresh nuts and seeds, and some types of fish are very good for you. The world's foremost expert on this matter is Dr. Udo Erasmus. I highly recommend the 'Udo's Oil' supplement for optimum cellular health.

Udo's Oil

Udo's Oil contains a 2-to-1 ratio of Omega 3 and Omega 6 fatty acids, which is crucial for good health. Diets high in omega-3 fatty acids and lower in omega-6 fatty acids can contribute to a decreased risk of heart disease, autoimmune diseases, breast cancer and colorectal cancer. Your body can't make essential fatty acids on its own (*hence the name essential!*), which makes them a crucial part of your daily diet. In addition to reducing the risk of certain health problems, **essential fatty acids also help repair your cell membranes, which enable them to absorb the nutrients from the foods you eat**. Healthy cell membranes also help remove toxins and waste from your body. In addition, fatty acids help your cells communicate with one another, so each of your bodily systems works properly.

Vitamin C - 500mg twice daily

Take as ascorbate; it will say Magnesium Ascorbate on the package which keeps the body alkaline - *not ascorbic acid*.

Vitamin C kills cancer cells while leaving normal cells alone. Dr. Linus Pauling and Dr. Ewan Cameron in 1976 reported that patients treated with high doses of vitamin C had survived three to four times longer than similar patients who did not receive vitamin C supplements. Studies show that intravenous vitamin C is the best protocol for destroying cancerous cells (this must be performed under the supervision of a doctor). The key is to be consistent with large quantities of vitamin C, taken several times every day. Vitamin C is a viable treatment for skin cancer. When vitamin C comes into contact with skin cancer, it hardens the tumor and forms a crust, such that the scab falls off in a couple of weeks or so. Scientists from India have demonstrated how the incidences of tumours of the breast in rats can be reduced by 88% by a single application of Magnesium Chloride, vitamin C, vitamin A, and Selenium.

Dr. Archie Kalokerinos in Australia found that children experiencing adverse reactions to vaccinations would recover after receiving large doses of vitamin C. The numbers of children who suffered adverse reactions declined dramatically when only healthy children who had taken large doses of vitamin C received vaccinations. Combining Echinacea and vitamin C reduced cold incidences by 86%, while Echinacea alone reduced colds by 65%.

A team of scientists from Arizona State University discovered that people with low blood concentrations of vitamin C burned 25% less fat during a 60-minute walk, compared with those who had adequate levels of vitamin C in their blood. The potential weight loss effects of vitamin C may be linked to the fact that it is needed for the production of Carnitine, a compound that encourages your body to turn fat into fuel, rather than store it as body fat.

The body benefits in many ways from taking Vitamin C, and never more than through the Peri-menopause stage of life. Vitamin C is a water soluble vitamin, which means that they are removed from the body easily through our kidneys, so are not stored in the body and must be replaced each day; hence the need to be taken twice daily.

Benefits of Vitamin C
The more we research Vitamin C, the more we realize its importance. There are too many known benefits to mention, but I have listed what I consider the big ones below:

- It's an important antioxidant - it prevents or slows down cell damage within the body.
- It's needed to produce and maintain a substance known as Collagen which:
    - Makes up to 90% of our bone matrix and is required to prevent Osteoporosis
    - Keeps skin and other soft tissues from drying out and withering up, such as the vaginal tissue - leading to painful intercourse; or bladder tissue - leading to stress incontinence
- We utilize a lot of our Vitamin C in times of stress so reducing your stress levels boosts your

Vitamin C.

- Vitamin C is essential to boost our immune system as a few components manufactured by the body to fight disease rely on it to perform effectively. When our levels are running low we leave our body wide open to developing lots of diseases.

- If we smoke or become stressed, our need for Vitamin C increases.

- Vitamin C is required to absorb Iron. Take the 2 supplements together to maximize the absorption of Iron.

- Studies on women taking Vitamin C in combination with bioflavonoids have shown reduction in hot flashes.

- Vitamin C neutralizes free radicals, which cause cell damage within the body.

- Vitamin C helps the body to reduce cholesterol and lowers blood pressure – high levels of both contribute to heart disease.

- Antioxidants of which Vitamin C is one – reduces the risk of developing Alzheimer's Disease.

- Vitamin C is required for Glucose metabolism – helping to regulate blood sugar levels.

- Your body burns calories more efficiently when vitamin C levels are raised.

- Vitamin C helps reduce excess levels of thyroid hormone in people with an over active thyroid gland.
- Maintains healthy hair.

Foods containing high amounts of Vitamin C include: citrus fruits (oranges, lemons and grapefruits), berries, green and leafy vegetables, tomatoes and green peppers.

Sometimes relying on food to get good amounts of vitamin C is difficult as Vitamin C is sensitive to light, air and heat, and can be easily destroyed by these.

When it comes to managing Menopause naturally, there is no 'one size fits all'. You need to find what combination works best for you. In addition to the recommendations to take a good quality multivitamin and mineral supplement, Omega 3 and 6, along with Vitamin C, I have outlined several other supplements recommended, and wildly used for managing the symptoms of Menopause. Based on the symptoms you find most debilitating, you can decide if you want to avail of the additional support of herbal remedies, and which ones will best suit your needs. I will give you the information required on the most commonly used herbs to help you make informed choices that best suit your requirements.

If you are already on hormone replacement therapy; hormonal contraceptives such as the Pill, the mini Pill, contraceptive injection, the coil or an implant; or if you are on hormonal medication such as anticancer treatments, caution is advised and consultation with your medical practitioner is recommended if you wish to consider starting any hormone-balancing herbs.

Black Cohosh
Recommended dose: 150 – 270mg per day

Black Cohosh is a herb which has been used for hundreds of years by the Native American Indian women. It has been the main herb of choice for many women seeking to steer clear of synthetic or chemical compounds used to treat the symptoms of Menopause. Black Cohosh works by mimicking the effect of the hormone Estrogen.

Black Cohosh is said to be a Selective Estrogen Receptor Modulator (SERM), which stimulates specific Estrogen receptors – only those in the bones and brain, while not having a stimulant effect on receptors in the womb or breasts. This is why it is considered safer than HRT in reducing the risk of cancers said to be Estrogen dependent (uterine and breast).

It is recommended to choose herbs that are not standardized as these are more natural, and are therefore similar to the way they would have been used traditionally. If it's possible, try to obtain organic varieties as these are best.

Black Cohosh may be your herb of choice (on its own or in combination with other supplements) if you are seeking relief from hot flashes, night sweats, anxiety, mood swings and/or depression.
It is certainly one of the most popular herbs used for the relief of hot flashes, and while the clinical trials conducted on it have not demonstrated a huge benefit when compared to placebo (dummy drug), the anecdotal evidence suggests it is of benefit to many Peri-menopausal women. It can be used in capsules or tincture (liquid) form.
As it is considered to have a beneficial effect on bone density due to its SERM activity stimulating Estrogen receptors in bones, if bone loss is of particular concern to you it is definitely worth considering.

Black Cohosh is considered the herb of choice if the primary symptoms are tiredness, low mood or sadness, lighter periods, and a longer time between periods.

Vitex Agnus Castus
Recommended dose: 300 – 550mg per day

Also called Vitex, Chaste tree, Chasteberry, Abraham's balm, Lilac Chastetree or Monk's pepper,
Vitex Agnus Castus is the fruit of the Chaste tree. It works on the body as an 'adaptogen.' This means it has a balancing effect on hormones, and works particularly well if your Progesterone levels are low, since it boosts production of your own Progesterone. This avoids the need to take synthetic Progesterone. It's known to be very effective when the main symptoms are anger, tension, anxiety or irritability, heavy periods and a short cycle (that is less than 26 days in the Peri-menopause phase).

Dong Quai
Recommended dose: 150 – 250mg per day

Dong Quai is also called Angelica Sinensis, Chinese angelica, female ginseng, or women's ginseng. It belongs to the carrot and celery plant family. The active ingredient is taken from the root of the plant, which has been used for thousands of years in Chinese, Korean and Japanese medicine.

155

The words Dong Quai actually translates as 'return to order' because of the herb's ability to promote overall body balancing and restoration. The plant is often referred to as women's ginseng due to the anecdotal reports (that is based on a person's experience) of its benefits to women's health. Used to successfully treat period pains, hot flashes, fatigue and low energy, it's also considered a strengthener of the heart, lungs, spleen, liver and kidneys, and a tonic for the blood.

If your sex hormones are not in balance you may experience low libido (sex drive). The good news is the adaptogenic effects of Dong Quai have been widely documented to be of great support to both men and women in this area.

Dong Quai is often used in combination with other herbs such as Agnus Castus to give the overall beneficial effect. There are very few studies in our western medicine into the uses of Dong Quai, but eastern medicine and women rely on the benefits they have gleaned from using it for centuries.

Dong Quai is not recommended for use by women with fibroids or blood-clotting disorders such as hemophilia, or if you're on Warfarin therapy, as it can interfere with the

156

clotting process in these circumstances.

Sage / Red sage
Recommended dose: 150 – 250mg per day

Sage (*Salvia officinalis*), is a member of the mint family. Most of us would be familiar with using Sage leaves in cooking, and it's these same leaves have been used by thousands of women for centuries for their therapeutic properties in treating Menopausal symptoms.

The most popular ways to take Sage is as a tea, or in capsule format. It is widely documented that Sage leaf is extremely helpful in reducing the severity and frequency of hot flashes and night sweats. Though not completely understood, this herb is unmistakably effective at regulating hormone imbalance. It has a positive influence on mood, and reduces stress and anxiety.

This combination of reduced sweating episodes coupled with the relaxing effect on the brain allows for better sleep and makes it an excellent natural remedy for Menopausal symptoms.

Homeopathy is based on the principle that a substance, which in large doses can produce a symptom, will cure that symptom when used in very small doses. For example, Sage essential oil is not recommended for use as it contains a substance called Thujone, which if taken in large amounts is toxic to the nervous system and may cause side effects or unwanted symptoms. On the other hand, the amount of Thujone found in sage tea or capsules is miniscule (compared to that in essential oil), and has great therapeutic calming effects on the brain, effectively treating anxiety, mood swings and memory difficulties.

Sage/Red sage is considered the herb of choice if the primary symptoms are hot flashes/night sweats, irregular and heavy uterine bleeding, or if you require a calming influence because of anxiety, restlessness or mood swings.

Milk Thistle (Silymarin Marianum)
Recommended dose: 140 milligrams three times per day for 3 weeks

The liver is one of the main processing plants in your body. It processes everything you eat and drink, all the nutrients as well as all the waste products, and toxins. So you can see the liver has a hugely important role, and its work is constant. As you go through life your liver is constantly striving to detoxify your body to maintain good health. During Menopause the liver comes under increased pressure due to the surge in hormone levels, as well as detoxifying the body if you make unhealthy food choices.

Milk thistle acts like a tonic on the liver and enhances its performance and detoxifying capabilities. This helps it to get rid for the excess Estrogen circulating though the body, reducing your Menopausal symptoms. This is especially beneficial to detoxify the body from Xenoestrogens (as mentioned in chapter 1), which are particularly harmful and are believed to contribute to hormone sensitive cancers (breast and uterine).

According to Phyllis D. Light, professor of herbal studies at Clayton College of Natural Health Birmingham, Alabama, all hormones produced by the body have to be metabolized by the liver. When the liver is congested, it becomes less efficient at breaking down neurotransmitters or stress hormones. Milk thistle was traditionally used as an herbal antidepressant; it works by increasing the efficiency of the liver, boosting its ability to process hormones and neurotransmitters. This makes it a good mood stabilizer and antidepressant, thereby reducing feelings of anxiety or depression.

Other symptoms of menopause alleviated by Milk thistle are fatigue, weight gain and constipation. In order for the body to work efficiently it needs the liver to be at the top of its game, which is particularly difficult if you are eating unhealthy foods (foods high in animal fat and refined carbohydrates). These foods clog up the liver, leaving it in overdrive trying to detoxify relentlessly. This has the knock on effect of reduced energy levels, and the liver then stores more fat, causing weight gain. Taking milk thistle, gives the liver the turbo-charge it needs to increase its efficiency, prevent fat storage and burn it up as fuel. Fluctuations in hormone levels reduce the production of bile (fluid produced by the liver to aid food digestion), this is the body's natural laxative, and when the liver is under pressure it produces less, leading to a sluggish digestive tract and constipation. Because Milk thistle is fat soluble, it should be taken with food.

Maca root (Lepidium Meyenii)
Recommended dose: Dependent on if it's powder or capsule consumed, see below

Similar to Vitex Agnus Castus, Maca is Phytoestrogen. It acts as an adaptogen, that is, it has a balancing effect on hormones. It stimulates and nourishes the hypothalamus and pituitary glands, which are the 'master glands' of the body. These glands then in turn have a balancing effect on the other glands in the body, including the adrenal glands and the pancreas. Maca is a member of the cruciferous family, the same as broccoli and cabbage, and is considered one of the super foods. It is rich in vitamins B, C and E, and also is naturally high in minerals (specifically Calcium, Potassium, Iron, Magnesium, Phosphorus and Zinc), as well as lots of other nutrients.

Due to its adaptability, it is often the first choice for many women looking to boost Estrogen levels naturally. Maca is widely used to promote sexual function of both men and women. It serves as a boost to your libido and increases endurance and at the same time it balances your hormones, relieves menstrual issues and Menopause. It alleviates cramps, body pain, hot flashes, anxiety, mood swings and depression. It is also known for increasing stamina and energy levels, which is why many athletes take Maca for peak performance. Maca supplies Iron and helps restore red blood cells, which aids anemia and cardiovascular diseases. Maca keeps your bones and teeth healthy and allows you to heal wounds more quickly. When used in conjunction with a good workout regime you will notice an increase in muscle mass. Many people take maca for skin issues; for some people it helps to clear acne and blemishes. If you find yourself overcome with anxiety, stress, depression or mood swings, Maca may help alleviate these symptoms. Some have also reported an increase in mental energy and focus.

Maca is relatively safe to take, but like any other supplement it should not be taken in large amounts. If you're new to Maca, start with small amounts and build up over days to allow your body and hormones time to adjust. If taking Maca powder - start with a small teaspoon per day and build up to 1 tablespoon (recommended daily dose). Maca also is available in capsule form, and I recommend following the manufacturer's instructions.

The more common side effects of Maca are hot flashes, extreme tiredness, abdominal cramps or headaches. While these can be confused with your normal Menopausal symptoms, if you find your usual symptoms worsening or you develop any of these side effects, then perhaps Maca is not the remedy for you.

Warning: If you are pregnant or lactating you should avoid taking Maca. Be cautious if you have a cancer related to hormones, like breast or ovarian. If you have liver issues or high blood pressure you should ask your doctor before taking Maca.

Ashwagandha
Recommended dose: 600 to 1,000 mg. twice daily
Ayurvedic medicine (also called Ayurveda) originated in India over 3,000 years ago, and is one of the world's oldest medical systems. The system promotes the use of herbal compounds in combination with specific diets to maintain good health and to treat medical conditions and diseases.

Ashwagandha is one of the herbs widely used in Ayurvedic medicine and is often referred to as "Indian ginseng" because of its rejuvenating properties; even though botanically, ginseng and Ashwagandha are unrelated. Ashwagandha is an herb with adaptogenic effects that modulate your response to stress or a changing environment. Adaptogens help the body cope with external stresses such as toxins in the environment and internal stresses such as anxiety and insomnia.

Ashwagandha acts on the endocrine system by encouraging hormone balance. A study involving 51 Menopausal women supplemented with Ashwagandha noted a significant reduction in symptoms such as hot flashes, anxiety and mood swings. Women taking Ashwagandha as a supplement also reported improved levels of concentration, memory and overall energy levels.

In her book "Herbal Medicine from the Heart of the Earth", Tilgner suggests that adults can take 10 to 60 drops of liquid extract three to four times per day in a little water or drink 1 cup of tea as many times daily. The recommended dose is 600 to 1000 milligrams twice daily, according to the Chopra Center website.

St. John's wort (botanical name Hypericum Perforatum)
Recommended dose: 300 mg twice a day

St. John's wort has long been used as a herbal anti-depressant, used instead of the pharmaceutical variety. St. John's wort is thought to work in a similar way as those prescribed by doctors, raising levels of serotonin (the happy hormone) in the brain. However the exact mechanism of action is not known. Due to its strong potency, it is not recommended to be used if you are already taking prescribed anti-depressants, and if you are interested in switching from the prescribed format to St John's Wort, this is best done in consultation with your doctor.

As well as improving your mood it has the added benefits of alleviating poor sleep, tiredness, anxiety and appetite changes.

American Skullcap (Scutellaria lateriflora)
Recommended dose: 10 drops of the tincture three times daily.

Skullcap is a flowering perennial plant from the mint family. It contains various phenolic compounds and flavones that impact the body in many different ways, and has been used traditionally by the Native-American for hundreds of years and remains in traditional use today.

Chinese skullcap is different to American skullcap, and so should be prepared in a very different way, so be sure you know which one you have. As we are aware, stress, anxiety and depressed mood can be some of the most debilitating symptoms of Menopause. Skullcap tea is a popular remedy to alleviate such symptoms. Skullcap rebalances hormones in your body, stimulates the release of endorphins, and generally balances your mood. If you are feeling tense for no reason, or experience a constant feeling of anxiety, then perhaps what you need is a cuppa. Phenolic compounds can have a wide range of effect on our hormonal balance, and Skullcap is rich in antioxidant properties. It might just be the remedy for you.

Now that you're familiar with the keys, and know how they work, you can start using them. I recommend implementing them all simultaneously, but if that all seems a little over-whelming, then take one or two at a time and get the hang of them, and then start on the next couple. The sooner you get started, the sooner you start to reap the benefits of a symptom-free and healthy life.

Chapter 9

Life After Menopause

During perimenopause and beyond, while we are experiencing the associated troublesome symptoms and trying desperately to get them under control, there may be other changes happening in our bodies that have little or no symptoms, and so can go undetected. Until one day it all comes to a head, and like a bolt out of the blue hits us like lightening, leaving us in a state of shock and exasperation!

As you know from reading about the functions of Estrogen and Progesterone (chapter 1), these hormones are responsible for a lot more going on in our bodies apart from reproduction. Therefore it's no surprise that when the hormone levels drop we experience the knock on effect, not just in our reproductive organs, but also all over the body, causing lots of upheaval to the previous status quo! I'm talking about the subtle changes going on in the body as we age that don't get any of our attention until we're diagnosed with it, such as:

167

- Osteoporosis
- Heart related problems such as;
    - High cholesterol (Hypercholesterolemia)
    - High blood pressure (Hypertension)
    - Heart disease
    - Stroke
- Breast cancer
- Vaginal or urinary issues

Osteoporosis

One of the major physiological effects of Estrogen is to slow down bone reabsorption, thereby helping the body to build up strong bones. With declining Estrogen levels during and after Menopause, the body finds it much harder to maintain bone strength. This makes us more susceptible to developing Osteoporosis; a condition where there is loss of bone density (thinning of the bones) putting us at risk of bone fractures or breaks. It is often called "the silent thief" because bone loss occurs without symptoms. It's estimated that 50% of women over the age of 50 will be diagnosed with Osteoporosis due to a rapid reduction in bone density as a result of Menopause.

It should be said that Menopause itself does not cause bone loss. Instead, the lack of Estrogen that signals the ovaries to stop producing eggs can lead to bone related issues. It's really important that we build up our bone strength prior to Menopause, and also actively work to maintain our bone density as we age.

While Menopause can be an indicator that women are at greater risk for developing bone loss, it is not the only indicator. Other indicators for bone loss besides menopause are:

- Being White or Asian
- If you had a premature menopause (before the age of 45) occurring naturally, or due to surgery or chemotherapy
- Regularly drinking coffee or black tea
- Regularly drinking alcohol (more than 7 units per week) - alcohol depletes your body of bone building nutrients
- Family history of Osteoporosis
- Inactive lifestyle
- Slim frame, or having anorexia
- Digestive problems such as lactose intolerance, coeliac, or Crohn's disease
- Low Vitamin D or Calcium Levels

- Being a current or previous smoker

Luckily it is often possible to prevent, delay or reduce bone loss through healthy living.

How do we avoid or manage it?

Stop Smoking

If you smoke - give it up! And avoid passive smoking, as both these can have a weakening effect on the bones. Through clinical studies they have identified that women who smoke tend to have lower Estrogen levels and therefore don't reap the same benefits of Estrogen in building strong bones compared with non-smokers. It's also thought that smokers reach Menopause earlier, and therefore bone density may also start to decline earlier than non-smokers.

Exercise

Regular weight bearing exercise such as fast-paced walking, jogging and resistance training also help to strengthen your bone structure. The World Health Organization (WHO) recommends a minimum of 150 minutes (2 ½ hours) of moderate-intensity aerobic activity per week. Aside from aerobic exercise, we should also do muscle-strengthening activities on two or more days a week by working all the major muscle groups, including the legs, hips, back, abdomen, chest, shoulders and arms.

Manage your stress

As mentioned previously, stress leads to high Cortisol levels which in turn have the knock on effect of:

- o Inhibiting bone building, while also causing bone to be resorbed faster into the blood stream.
- o Decreasing mineral absorption in the gut - so you won't be absorbing the calcium and magnesium required to build bone
- o Increasing kidney output, spilling out calcium from the body

Get yourself a Dexa Scan (bone density scan), to see what is your level of bone density currently is, and then you have a baseline to work from.

This is another good reason to keep stress levels low, so please consider the recommendations offered in Key No. 4: *Sleep & De-stress.*

Health Eating

Calcium is one of our essential minerals. In addition to building and maintaining bone health, Calcium also

171

helps our blood clotting mechanism, our nervous system and our muscles to work efficiently. About 99% of the Calcium in our bodies is in our bones and teeth. Each day we lose Calcium through our skin, nails, hair, sweat, urine and feces, and our bodies cannot produce new calcium. This is why it's so important to get calcium from the food we eat. When we don't get enough calcium for our body's needs, it is taken from our bones.

If you haven't already taken on the recommendations in *Key No. 1: The food we eat* (chapter 3), you'll need to start so that your body is getting Calcium through your diet, which will reduce the effects of low Estrogen on your bones. Foods high in Calcium include dark leafy greens vegetables, broccoli, green beans and bok-choy, almonds, sesame seeds, oranges, figs and oily fish such as sardines and salmon.

There is currently a lot of controversy and debate on the alkalinity of the blood in relation to bone health. When the body is more alkaline, the body is better able to absorb Calcium and utilize it for bone health. When the body is acidic (the opposite to alkaline) it is thought that the body loses Calcium from bone because it is used to rebalance the body's pH balance, bringing it back to an alkaline state. An alkaline diet is essentially a

172

healthy diet – high in fruit and vegetables and low in processed foods, dairy and wheat. Therefore by following the recommendations in chapter 3, while it is not an alkaline diet in the strict sense of the word, it will provide a healthy pH balance, and one that is also high in Calcium.

Foods to avoid

Caffeine, sugar and alcohol. Assuming you've taken on the recommendations I made earlier in the book (Key No. 1 & 3) of reducing or quitting caffeine, sugar and alcohol to gain significant improvements in symptoms of Menopause, you will reap the additional reward of improving your bone density. If you haven't managed to at least reduce, or better again quit these, here's another reason to give these toxic substances up: Cola drinks have been shown through clinical trials to have an adverse effect on Calcium absorption and should be eliminated completely.

Supplements

- **Calcium (500mg Calcium Citrate)**
  When taking a Calcium supplement, it's best taken in combination with Magnesium and vitamin D3 (Cholecalciferol), which aid absorption of calcium.

173

If you have children, especially girls, ensure that they keep their Vitamin D3 and Calcium at optimal levels throughout their development. A woman usually has her most dense bones at about age 30, so if you build until then, you're going to lower your risk of Osteoporosis substantially.

- **Vitamin D3 Cholecalciferol (1,000 IU daily)**
Research continues to accumulate documenting Cholecalciferol's role in the reduction of the risk of fractures to a significant degree. Vitamin D3 is the only vitamin the body can manufacture from sunlight (UVB). Yet with today's indoor living and extensive use of sunscreen due to concern about skin cancer, we are now more susceptible to becoming deficient in vitamin D3, unless we live near the equator. The Recommended Daily Intake (RDI) of Vitamin D3 is set at 400 to 800 International Units (I.U.) in most developed countries. Researchers working extensively on Vitamin D3 now feel that this is a sub-optimal level. For example, an analysis of the medical literature found that at least 1,000 to 2,000 IU of

Vitamin D3 per day is necessary to reduce the risk of colorectal cancer and that lower doses of Vitamin D3 did not have the same protective effect.

- **Vitamin B complex**

  Just as Vitamin B complex is good to reduce the symptoms of Menopause, it has also been shown to help reduce the levels of Homocysteine. Homocysteine is an amino acid produced in the body as part of protein metabolism. It's believed that high levels of Homocysteine in our blood causes inflammation and contributes to a large number of preventable diseases including Osteoporosis, memory loss, coronary artery disease, high cholesterol, blood clots, heart attacks and strokes. We can maintain lower Homocysteine levels by following the recommendations in Key No. 1: Food.

- **Probiotics**

  These are healthy bacteria found in our digestive tract. Aside from stopping the 'bad' bacteria from taking hold which cause infection, probiotic bacteria have other beneficial uses, especially for our bones. A healthy probiotic balance improves bone health by increasing our absorption of Calcium and Magnesium, and also reduces the impact of Phytates, which can limit absorption of minerals including Iron, Zinc, Manganese and, to a lesser extent, Calcium. Probiotics also increase the absorption of Vitamin K2 which has been shown through clinical studies to aid the deposit of Calcium in appropriate locations, such as in the bones and teeth, and prevents it from depositing in locations where it does not belong, such as the soft tissues.

- **Magnesium**
  This is one of our essential nutrients and has many functions in the body. Most notably, adequate Magnesium is essential for absorption and metabolism of Calcium and vitamin D. So even if we are taking in adequate amounts of calcium and vitamin D, if our Magnesium is low, the Calcium and vitamin D is of little use to us. Magnesium is stored in the bones, so if we

become deficient in Magnesium, we take it from our bones to use, making our bones weaker and leading to Osteoporosis.

- **Zinc (Recommended supplement 15mgs daily)**
  A little known mineral found in many foods, Zinc is required by the body to help osteoblasts (bone building cells) do their bone-building work. Zinc is also crucial for Vitamin D to get into cells where it can work to build bones. Zinc can also be found in components of bone, which makes up about half of our bones' weight.

- **Boron (Recommended supplement 3mgs daily)**
  The body requires boron for proper metabolism and utilization of various bone-building substances, including Calcium, Magnesium, vitamin D and Estrogen.

It is possible to get good quality supplements which contain a combination of the vitamins and minerals listed above, so that rather than taking a few tablets, they are all contained in one.

Avoid   Unnecessary   Medications: Steroids, diuretics, antacids, and even hormone replacement medications are some of the medications that can increase the rate of bone loss. If you have been prescribed any of these by your doctor, do not stop the medication without prior consultation with them, but do discuss it with them to see if there are better alternatives.

Menopause-related bone loss doesn't have to happen if you take care of yourself, exercise and eat right. But since Menopause is a natural state that will happen with every woman who lives long enough, it's important to concentrate on being healthy throughout your life to avoid this potentially damaging side effect. Eat right, exercise and take good general care of yourself and you will keep your bones healthy.

Heart disease & Stroke

As we mentioned in chapter 1, some of the functions of Estrogen include:

- ✓ Increases   HDL   (good   cholesterol)   and triglycerides,   and   decreases   LDL   (bad cholesterol)
- ✓ Influences salt and water retention, affecting blood pressure

✓ Helps with the blood clotting mechanism
✓ Increases collagen content and quality, which keeps elasticity in connective tissues including our arteries. Estrogen is believed to have a positive effect on the inner layer of the artery walls, helping to keep blood vessels flexible. That means they can relax and expand to accommodate blood flow, and maintain good blood pressure.

The two biggest health issues to concern women after Menopause are Osteoporosis and Coronary Heart Disease (CHD). Heart disease is the number 1 killer of women across most countries of the world. We can see from the list of effects Estrogen has relating to the functions of our heart, that it's no surprise that we are prone to develop heart issues after Menopause when our Estrogen levels fall. The risk of heart disease rises for all of us as we age, but understandably for women symptoms can become more evident after the onset of Menopause.

Menopause does not cause Coronary Heart Disease. However, certain risk factors such as unhealthy food habits, excess weight (especially around our waist area), lack of exercise and smoking, in *combination* with Menopause increase our incidence dramatically. We

179

may have 'got away with' the other risk factors up until Menopause, but they start to take their toll in the absence of Estrogen, and like the 'house of cards', when one thing starts to go wrong for us, the slippery slope to ill-health can be hard to stop, and the house of cards (our body) comes tumbling down!

Coronary Heart Disease (CHD) is a condition where a sludge-like substance builds up, called 'plaque' inside the artery walls (arteries carry oxygen rich blood around the body from the heart). Over time as the plaque builds up, the inside of the arteries become narrow, making it harder for the blood to flow through - this is called atherosclerosis. As we mentioned above, one of the functions of Estrogen is to keep the blood vessels flexible; so when Menopause occurs and Estrogen drops, the arteries become harder and inflexible contributing to the problem. Now we have inflexible and narrowed arteries, the blood pressure rises. When the plaque ruptures, a blood clot forms and this partially or completely blocks blood flow through an artery supplying the heart itself; the most common cause of heart attacks.

A stroke is sometimes called a 'brain attack', as it is the same process that occurs in the body as a heart attack, except it occurs in one of the blood vessels in the brain.

The primary cause of heart disease is not high cholesterol or high blood pressure; these are also symptoms of the same cause – Inflammation. Inflammation under normal circumstances is good, like when we sprain an ankle, it becomes inflamed, stopping us from using it until the body has had a chance to heal itself. The real concern is the chronic, smoldering inflammation that slowly destroys our organs (including the heart) and our ability to function well and leads to rapid aging. The most common causes of inflammation are poor diet—mostly sugar, refined carbohydrates, processed foods, trans fats and saturated fats - lack of exercise and stress.

How do we avoid or manage it?

All of the keys I have given you in this book to become free from Menopause will also go a long way towards preventing the onset of high blood pressure, atherosclerosis, heart disease or stroke.

Sugar, or more accurately put, refined carbohydrates are the cause of a lot of our health issues. As I explained in chapter 3, when you eat refined carbohydrates such as white bread, blood sugar rises quickly, causing the brain to signal the pancreas to produce extra insulin (the hormone that controls your blood sugar). Insulin helps take sugar out of your blood, usually by converting the excess sugar into fat and storing it in your body. High levels of insulin create free radicals and also stimulate the liver to produce more cholesterol (a normal function of the liver). The free radicals in turn work on fats, causing them to break down and form plaques on the arteries

Normally, the body can handle free radicals, but if antioxidants are unavailable, or if the free-radical production becomes excessive, damage ensues. Of particular importance is that free radical damage accumulates with age. Prolonged excessive insulin secretion results in various ill health effects such as high blood pressure, high cholesterol, weight gain and eventually, heart disease. Do yourself a huge favor and take on the tips for healthy eating in chapter 3.

Exercise
When it comes to exercise, we have lots of evidence to demonstrate that regular exercise reduces inflammation. It also has the added benefits of improving immune function, strengthening your cardiovascular system, improving Glucose metabolism and improving our mood.

According to the World Health Organization (WHO), exercising 30 minutes a day, five days a week will improve your heart health and help reduce your risk of heart disease. You can even break it up into quick and manageable 10-minute sessions, three times a day. So get going!

Stress management

Learn how to relax, and practice it regularly. Look back to the tips I gave in Key No. 4: *Sleep and De-stress*. When you learn how to relax your whole body it helps to lower inflammation. Practice Yoga or meditation, breathe deeply, or even take a warm bath to help you chill out!

Supplements

As previously, I recommend taking a multivitamin, a multi-mineral supplement, Omega 3 rich fish oil and vitamin D for Menopausal symptoms, as all of these also help reduce inflammation. Take probiotics too to help your digestion and improve the balance of healthy bacteria in your gut to also reduce inflammation.

There is a genetic predisposition to heart disease, and lots of people think, '*Oh well my mother or father had heart disease, so I'll probably get it too*', when nothing could be further from the truth. If a member of your family has been previously diagnosed with heart disease or stroke, then yes you are at a higher risk of developing the same. However this is all the more motivation to take exceptional care to ensure you don't end up the same way. All of these conditions are called lifestyle diseases because they are caused by the lifestyles we lead. If we make some healthy choices about the food we eat, exercise, stress management and taking appropriate supplements, we're choosing to live a healthy and fulfilling life.

Breast cancer

According to the World Cancer Research Fund (WCRF), Breast cancer is the most common cancer in women worldwide, with nearly 1.7 million new cases diagnosed in 2012 (the second most common cancer overall). This represents about 12% of all new cancer cases and 25% of all cancers in women.

Breast cancer is hormone related, and the factors that modify the risk of this cancer when diagnosed prior to menopause and when diagnosed post-menopause (more prevalent) are not the same.

The Continuous Update Project Panel from the WCRF judged that for Post-menopausal breast cancer, there was convincing evidence that consuming alcoholic drinks, body fatness and *adult attained height, increase the risk of this cancer, and if you had breast fed in the past this protects against it. Abdominal fatness and adult weight gain are probably causes of this cancer and physical activity probably protects against it.

Taller people have a greater chance of developing cancer than shorter people; however the reason for this is unclear

How do we avoid or manage it?

The Continuous Update Project Panel identified 10 cancer prevention recommendations that reduce the risk of developing cancer, 3 of which are specific to Breast Cancer:

1. **Drinking alcohol** - For cancer prevention, it's best not to drink alcohol, or limit it to one per day for women or two per day for men. Alcohol is also a risk factor for bowel, liver, mouth, larynx and esophageal cancers. As said previously, you may have reduced your alcoholic intake to become free from Menopausal symptoms, so here's another good reason for taking this healthy step.

2. **Physically active** – Be moderately physically active, equivalent to brisk walking, for at least 30 minutes every day. As fitness improves, aim for 60 minutes or more of moderate, or 30 minutes or more of vigorous physical activity every day. Limit sedentary habits such as watching television

3. **Maintain a healthy weight** - Through a balanced diet and regular physical activity. This helps reduce the risk of developing cancer. It's recommended to be as lean as possible within the normal range of body weight.

4. **Take supplements** - to support your good work. As previously recommended, take a good multivitamin and multi-mineral as well as Omega 3 fish oil. A review of 63 observational studies *(published in the Am J of Public Health)*, looked at Vitamin D levels and incidence of cancers; the majority of studies found a protective relationship between sufficient vitamin D status and lower risk of cancer. The evidence suggests that efforts to improve vitamin D status, for example by vitamin D supplementation, could reduce cancer incidence

and mortality at low cost, with few or no adverse effects. Hopefully by now you are taking Vitamin D to enhance your bone health, and reaping the additional benefit of protection against multiple cancers. The recommended dose is 1,000 – 2,000 IU per day.

Vaginal or urinary issues

Unlike the other conditions mentioned in this chapter, which all come about relatively symptom free, it's the symptoms and associated discomfort around Vaginal or urinary issues that prompt us to take action.

Before Menopause, the skin and tissues around the vagina are kept supple and moist by fluids and mucus. Estrogen stimulates glands at the neck of the womb to produce these fluids and mucus. Estrogen also affects the tissues in and around the vagina, causing the lining of the vagina to be thicker and more elastic. Estrogen also stimulates the cells that line the vagina to produce a substance called Glycogen, which encourages the presence of helpful germs (bacteria) to protect the vagina from infections.

In the absence of Estrogen, during the Peri-menopause and Post-menopause stages of life, the lack of Estrogen leads to thinning of the tissues around the vagina and a reduction in the number of glands that make mucus, causing the vagina to become shorter, less elastic and drier. This change occurs over time, often taking years to see a noticeable difference, and is medically called 'Atrophic Vaginitis'. This condition can create great physical discomfort such as:

- **Discomfort** - if the vulva or vagina is sore and red
- **Pain during sex** - this may occur because the vagina is smaller, drier and less likely to become lubricated during sex. Also, the skin around the vagina is more fragile and with friction can become painful and even bleed, putting some women off sex completely. This puts pressure on the relationship with their loved one, and adds to the stress in their lives.
- **Vaginal discharge** - As the area is no longer protected by glycogen, women are now more prone to developing infections in this area. There may be a white or yellow discharge which is sometimes due to an infection. Infection is more likely if the discharge has an unpleasant smell.
- **Itchy** - the skin around the vagina becomes more sensitive and more likely to itch. It can be very

difficult not to scratch to relive the itch, however this makes the area even more irritated and itchy, causing an itch/scratch cycle which can be difficult to break and can be very uncomfortable.

- **Urinary problems** – reduced levels of Estrogen cause thinning and weakening of the tissues around the opening to the bladder (urethra), causing 'urinary urgency' (urgency to get to the toilet on time) and recurring urinary tract infections, often medically referred to as UTI's.

How do we avoid or manage it?
Avoid all harsh, scented and chemical based soaps in the vaginal area. This will destroy the natural pH balance of the vagina. Vaginal douching is also not recommended. Use only unscented and pH balancing products in the vaginal area to maintain the pH balance and avoid irritation.

Multivitamin & Multi-mineral Supplements
As previously recommended, take a good multivitamin and multi-mineral supplement.

Omega 3
Foods that are very high in omega 3 fatty acids are good for increasing vaginal lubrication. This would

include sunflower seeds, raw pumpkin, sesame seeds and oily fish such as tuna, mackerel or salmon are especially good to reduce the dryness from the inside out.

Vitamin C

The body uses vitamin C to produce collagen, which in turn maintains flexibility in the vaginal wall, reducing the discomfort. The collagen maintains flexibility in the wall of the urethra (entry to the bladder), reducing the risk of urinary tract infections.

Probiotics

With the change in the pH balance within the vagina, it's important to have good levels of beneficial bacteria by taking a probiotic regularly. It boosts the good bacteria in the gut and reduces the incidence of developing vaginal thrush or other vaginal and urinary infections.

Natural Lubricant

If vaginal dryness is a specific problem for you, lubricating gels may help. There are different lubricants which can work well to improve the dryness during sexual intercourse. These include a few natural options like aloe, or Sylk®, Yes® and Good Clean Love®. You can buy all of these online. They are all natural lubricants and are certified organic, guaranteed pure &

natural and are free from Parabens or Glycerine.

Cranberries

Inflammation of the bladder (medically called Cystitis), can be a very uncomfortable and painful condition causing such symptoms as:

- A strong, persistent feeling that you need to pee (called urinary urgency)
- A burning sensation when passing urine
- Going to the toilet frequently but only passing small amounts (called urinary frequency)
- Occasionally blood in the urine (hematuria)
- Pain or discomfort in the bladder or pelvic area
- A feeling of pressure in the lower abdomen
- Occasionally a low-grade fever

Most of the time the inflammation is caused by a bacterial infection, less commonly, cystitis may occur as a reaction to certain drugs, radiation therapy or potential irritants such as feminine hygiene spray or spermicidal jellies. The usual treatment for bacterial cystitis is a course of antibiotics. It's relatively common for post-menopausal women to suffer from recurrent cystitis.

Clinical trials have demonstrated that cranberries prevent bacteria from sticking to the bladder wall, thereby preventing the bacteria from taking hold and

191

causing infection. Cranberry can be taken as an unsweetened drink, or in capsule form.

Cranberry extract tablets: 1 tablet (800mg)
Take three times per day while you have a UTI, or once daily if there is no infection present. If taking the unsweetened juice: take 8 oz / 250mls three times daily.

I know from reading this last chapter you're probably wondering if is there any good news to aging! The good news is that we are unique. We're not all susceptible to all the conditions mentioned here, and the better we are at maintaining overall health, the less likely we are to suffer from any of these.

It's also important to note that as we are unique, we respond differently to different remedies. What works great for your best friend who's advised you, may not necessarily work for you, so see for yourself what the best keys are to unlock your freedom to great health. No matter what, using the keys given to you here; eating well, exercising, sleeping well and taking good care of yourself, among others, will help you to master the Menopause naturally, leading to great health and giving you the freedom to embrace and enjoy your life.

Take Care

Appendix

List of foods classified as refined carbohydrates (this list is not exhaustive):

- All white and brown breads unless they say '100% whole-wheat' or 'whole-grain' (these are not refined)
- Breaded or battered foods and croutons
- All types of dough or pastry, bagels, pretzels
- Most cereals, except 100% whole grain cereals in which you can see the whole grains in their entirety with the naked eye (unsweetened muesli, rolled oats, or unsweetened puffed grain cereals are good examples)
- Most pastas, noodles and couscous
- Most desserts including cakes, muffins, pancakes, waffles, pies and pastries, puddings and custards
- Sweetened yogurts and other sweetened dairy products, ice cream, sherbet and frozen yogurt
- Most crackers, biscuits and sweets
- All chocolate (dark, milk and white), including that used in baking
- Jellies, jams and preserves
- Pizza (because of the flour in the dough)
- Corn chips, Tortillas (unless 100% stone-ground whole grain)

- Most muesli bars, power bars, energy bars, etc. - unless labeled sugar-free, or low GI (glycemic index)
- Most rice cakes and corn cakes (except the 100% whole grain ones)
- Sauces such as Ketchup, honey mustard, barbecue salsa, tomato sauces, salad dressings and other jarred/canned sauces unless it says sugar free
- Honey-roasted nuts
- Sweetened sodas
- Condensed milk
- Most milk substitutes (almond milk, soy milk, oat milk, etc.) as often there is sugar added - check the food label
- Sweet wines and liqueurs

Examples of Saturated Fats	Examples of Polyunsaturated Fats
Limit your intake of these	Considered better for your health
Hydrogenated Oils (Palm Oil)	
Dairy Butter and cream	Soybeans and Soybean oil
Cocoa Butter	Corn oil
	Sunflower seeds and Sunflower oil
Light Butter	Fatty fish such as salmon, mackerel, herring and trout
Whipped Butter	Walnuts
Animal fats, including Tallow	
Meat Drippings	Flaxseed (AKA Linseed)
Shortening	Tofu
Lard, Duck Fat and Goose Fat	
	Contain both Saturated and Polyunsaturated Fats
Milk Chocolate	
All dairy cheese	All parts of the coconut
Processed Meats, Bacon, Pork Sausage,	Wheat Germ & Oat Oils (Wheat Germ Oil)
Italian Salami, Salami & Frankfurter	Sesame Oil
Luncheon Meat and Chorizo	Olive Oil
Doughnuts, Cakes and Pies	Nuts and seeds
Croissants	Dark Chocolate
Potato Chips (Crisps)	Oily Fish & Fish Oils (Mackerel)
Fast Food	Avocado Oil
Biscuits	Peanut Butter
Patties & Burgers	

Anti-Oxidant Rich foods

Blackberries

Blueberries

Cranberries

Raspberries

Strawberries

Cloves

Pecan nuts

Walnuts

Artichoke hearts

Red or black grapes

Dark green veg - broccoli, spinach and Kale

Leeks, lettuce

Sweet potato

Carrots

Black tea (preferably caffeine free)

Green tea

Whole grain bread

Wild or brown rice

Corn tortillas

www.ingramcontent.com/pod-product-compliance
Lightning Source LLC
Chambersburg PA
CBHW071743270326
41928CB00013B/2779